Low
Vision
Care

Low Vision Care

by
EDWIN B. MEHR, O.D., F.A.A.O.
and
ALLAN N. FREID, M. OPT., O.D., F.A.A.O.

School of Optometry
University of California
Berkeley, California

The Professional Press, Inc.
Chicago, Illinois

© 1975 by Professional Press, Inc.

FIRST PRINTING
ISBN-0-87873-016-8

Library of Congress Catalog Card Number: 74-17532

Published by Professional Press, Inc.
Chicago, Illinois 60611

Printed in the U.S.A.

Dedicated to
WILLIAM FEINBLOOM, O.D., PH.D.
and
MEREDITH MORGAN, JR., O.D., PH.D.

Preface

In 1960 the American Academy of Optometry met in San Francisco. The authors enrolled in a six hour course by William Feinbloom on Subnormal Vision. An eight-year-old girl who was being educated in Braille met the master clinician and read 6 point type! It probably changed her life. We did not realize it at the time, but that course had changed our professional lives.

We had read the classic I H B Optical Aids Service Survey published in 1957. We tried fitting low vision patients. Our successes were the exceptions, our failures memorable. We realized it could be done. It had been done, but we didn't have the secret.

Now, in 1960, we knew how to do it. More than that we felt an obligation to help our colleagues take care of the neglected low vision population.

There followed seminars on care of the partially-sighted for our own optometric society. This led to invitations to present lectures and courses before alumni groups, other optometric societies, state congresses, A.O.A. congresses, and the American Academy of Optometry. We became involved in committees for aid to the partially-sighted at state and national levels.

Over the years more and more partially-sighted patients found their way to our offices and we had the opportunity to work as part of a multi-disciplinary team at the Vision Rehabilitation Center of Santa Clara County. We had the opportunity to see numerous patients as chiefs of the Low Vision Clinic at the School of Optometry at the University of California. As consultant to the Western Blind Rehabiliation Center of the Veterans Administration another multi-disciplinary opportunity was available.

Dean Meredith Morgan is the man responsible for our writing this book. He originally suggested it; he read chapters as we produced them, offered suggestions and encouragement. We owe him a great debt of thanks.

Others at the University have been helpful with suggestions and reviewing specific areas. In this respect we especially wish to thank Anthony Adams and Robert Mandell.

The chapter on Psychological and Sociological Factors was written in collaboration with Helen M. Mehr, who also contributed to discussions pertaining to psychology in other chapters. Suggestions relating to discussions of psychology were also made by Harriett Turner.

The index was expertly prepared by Grace Weiner.

Illustrations were produced by the Multimedia Department of the School of Optometry with the able assistance of Bob Tarr. Drafting was ably performed by Gloria Petrowski. Typing was done by Sharon Godske, Irene Thomas, Patricia Olson, Sara McManis, Margaret Payne, Lindale Zilliox, Diane Dobbins and Bea Keller.

To all these people we owe thanks. We also owe a debt of gratitude to all our colleagues in the low vision field who generously shared their ideas and experiences with us. The biggest debt is owed to our patients. They provided the questions, the challenges, and often the answers.

EDWIN B. MEHR
ALLAN N. FREID

Table of Contents

Chapter 1

Introduction

Definition

Low vision, partial sight, or *subnormal vision* may be defined as reduced central acuity or visual field loss which even with the best optical correction provided by regular lenses still results in visual impairment from a performance standpoint.

There are certain things generally assumed by this definition:

1) That the vision loss is bilateral.
2) That some form vision remains.
3) That "regular lenses" do not include reading adds over $+4.00$ D., telescopes, pinholes, visors, or other "unusual" devices which will be categorized as *low vision aids.*

Limits

Visual acuity is not the best criterion—impairment of performance is the ultimate criterion. However, since this is not easily quantified, we communicate better when we use visual acuity. It is generally agreed that an acuity of 20/70 or poorer (for the better eye) with corrective lenses constitutes low vision. Where other factors also cause limitations of vision (e.g. field losses), a person may be so classified even with 20/20 acuity.

If we think in terms of using low vision aids to improve the visual performance, the lower limit is dependent on many factors besides visual acuity. Where acuity is better than 20/600 the chances of helping the patient optometrically are excellent. When the corrected visual acuity is 20/2000 or poorer the chances of this kind of help are almost nil.

Prevalence

Statistics regarding prevalence of blindness are inadequate. With respect to the group that is partially-sighted, but not legally blind, accurate figures are almost *totally* lacking. Based on these poor statistics, we can only make educated guesses.

Brazelton (1964) estimated the numbers conservatively at 5-10/1000. Among school children it has been estimated by the National Society for the Prevention of Blindness (1961) that at least 1/500 are partially-sighted. Even among the legally *blind* children (20/200 or less V.A. - or field of 20° or less), 60% had *useful residual* vision as reported by the U.S. Department of Health, Education and Welfare (1961).

U.S. Department of HEW reports on those on blind registers in the model reporting area for 1970 (Kahn and Moorhead, 1973) a record 161.7/100,000 population. This starts with 10.0/100,000 for those under 5 years of age rising steadily to 200.7/100,000 for the 45 to 64 age group. Prevalence rises rapidly to 2621.1/100,000 in the 85 years and over group. While these figures may indicate the relative distribution of blind by age group, they do not reflect the true totals in the population, since many (and we can only guess how many) of the legally blind never get on the *official* register. Using a household interview survey, the National Health Survey reported the prevalence of severe visual impairment in both eyes "as four times the model reporting area figures for reported legal blindness". [Riley, 1969])

Between 71% and 77% of the legally blind had recorded form vision. Hence the major portion even of those classified as blind should be treated clinically as partially-sighted.

No attempt is even made to register the group that is partially-sighted but not legally blind. Goldish and Marx (1973) estimate the U.S. partially-sighted at 6 million, including 1.3 million functioning as legally blind. Genensky (1973), using a conservative approach, estimates the number of U.S. partially-sighted at slightly over 1.6 million. He extrapolates this conservative figure to the world population to conclude that there are at least 30 million partially-sighted people in the world.

Need

There is a great unmet need for good vision care for the partially-sighted population. Even in an advanced and affluent country like the U.S., the majority of the partially-sighted have never had an adequate low vision examination. Possibly 15% of those who could benefit from low vision aids have had them prescribed. Rosenbloom (1970) estimates the group that can be helped by reading aids as 1,000,000.

Some of the more enterprising and determined partially-sighted patients have discovered aids by themselves in camera shops, hobby shops, variety stores, etc. While of some assistance, these chance selected aids are usually far from adequate for their needs. But these patients were unwilling to accept the dicta of their ophthalmologists or optometrists that "nothing more can be done", or "you have the strongest lenses I can give you".

Monroe Hirsch (1964) has said: "We have, then, a situation where people—many people—can be helped who are now being cast aside. And this situation exists only because of lack of knowledge—by optometrists, by ophthalmologists, by laymen, by social workers, and by agencies which could help if they knew better."

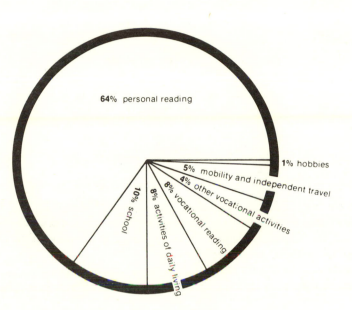

Fig. I-1.   Primary objectives of low vision care patients (Goldish and Marx, 1973). Reproduced by permission of The New Outlook For The Blind.

Goldish and Marx (1973) surveyed the primary objectives of low vision care patients. They reported that for two out of three, the principle objective was a desire to read personal materials (see Figure I-1).

Historical Background

Some form of low vision aid has been available for many years. Simple magnifying lenses were known before spectacles. Stenopaic spectacles have been used for at least 300 years. The typoscope was described by Charles Prentice in 1897 (Prentice and Mehr, 1969).

The twentieth century has seen the contributions of von Rohr, Feinbloom, Policoff, Ellerbrock, Bechtold, Kestenbaum, Lederer, Hoff, Faye, Fonda, Keeler, Bier, Hellinger, Sloan, Genensky, and many others in developing lens systems and clinical techniques to aid the partially-sighted.

Along with these scientific developments has gone a slow change in attitude by the professions. Where previously patients had been advised to "save" their sight, they are now encouraged to use their remaining vision as fully as possible.

The current trends in this field are to integrate the blind into the sighted population, and to emphasize the positive. It is in line with this attitude that the positive term *partially-sighted* is preferred to *partially-blind*. Likewise, *low vision* does not imply the undesirable connotations of *subnormal vision*.

Types of Aids

At one time the pioneers in the field of "subnormal vision" were concentrating on the telescopic spectacle as a new and promising departure. Because of their complexities, and the different techniques involved in the use of telescopes, much time in courses on low vision may be devoted to telescopic spectacles.

Consequently, many optometrists have for years thought of "subnormal vision" care as synonymous with fitting telescopic spectacles.

The facts are very much the opposite. The Industrial Home for the Blind (1957) analysis of 500 cases showed only 11.6% of the aids prescribed were telescopics. Rosenbloom (1966) reporting on 1,000 cases at the Chicago Lighthouse said, "Telescopic lenses, often of the ready-made type, were prescribed in about 10 percent of the cases".

The Industrial Home for the Blind Survey classified their aids prescribed as follows:

Near Vision Spectacles	29%	⎫
Distance Vision Spectacles	26.7%	⎬ 68.8%
Bifocal Spectacles	13.1%	⎭
Microscopics	10.9%	
Microscopic Bifocals	2.9%	
Telescopics	10.9%	
3.5× Sportoculars	0.7%	
Contact Lenses	0.6%	
Auxiliary Aids	5.2%	

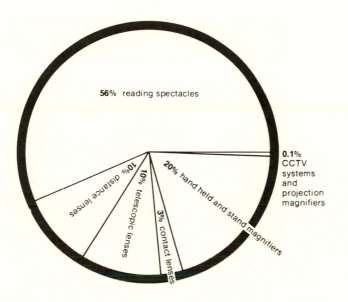

Fig. I-2.   Types of aids prescribed by low vision clinics (Goldish and Marx, 1973). Reproduced by permission of The New Outlook For The Blind.

Sixteen years later, Goldish and Marx (1973) surveyed a group of low vision clinics and found a similar pattern of aids prescribed. The main difference being a greater use of hand held and stand magnifiers by the surveyed clinics (Figure I-2).

The startling fact in the Industrial Home for The Blind study is that *ordinary* lenses, of the type that any competent ophthalmic laboratory should be able to supply and which could be prescribed from any *ordinary* trial lens set, accounted for almost 69% of the aids they prescribed! The authors heartily agree with their conclusion "that it is the technique of the low vision examination rather than the use of unusual lenses, which in the majority of these cases is responsible for the favorable results".

Chapter 2

Identifying the Successful Low Vision Patient

General

There is an implication in the title of this chapter that there *are* successful low vision patients. Many optometrists and ophthalmologists have acted and spoken as though they doubted this.

How Many Can Be Helped?

Survey Results

Various studies in recent years have published surprisingly similar figures.

A. The Industrial Home for the Blind (1957), New York, survey by George Hellinger, O. D. et al., reported only on legally blind (N = 500).

    1. 68% benefitted by aids

    2. 14% could have benefitted, but didn't adapt

    3. 18% couldn't be helped in the opinion of the examiner

B. Maryland Workshop for the Blind, survey by Robert E. Schwartz, O. D. (1960) (N = 500).

    1. 74.8% could be helped

C. Chicago Lighthouse for the Blind, survey by Alfred A. Rosenbloom, Jr., O. D. (1966) (N = 1800).

    68% benefitted

2. 7% could have benefitted, but did not adapt

D. It should be noted that these figures are almost entirely for legally blind patients. There is every reason to believe that the figures for the group with reduced vision, not severe enough to be classified as blind, would be even more favorable.

Ellerbrock (1960) has stated the case very succinctly when he said:

> "It is a rule rather than an exception that partial vision, especially at near distance, can be improved with optical aids."

Prognostic Factors

The factors that determine the success potential of a particular patient are interrelated, however, we may itemize some of them as in the following table:

Prognosis Table

Factor	Good Prognosis	Poor Prognosis	Comments
A. Visual acuity	A. 20/70 to 20/600	A. Too low (below 20/2000)	A. There is obviously a group falling between acuities of 20/600 and 20/2000 who have neither a very good nor a very poor prognosis.
B. Duration	B. Vision loss over five years (includes all congenitals)	B. Very recent vision loss (still looking for a cure)	B. All recent vision losses are not poor risks. A person who is highly motivated to earn a living or continue in school may be a very good patient despite a very recent loss, if he has accepted the fact of his loss and realizes that he must organize his life around it.
C. Motivation	C. Highly motivated to do something where performance can be improved by an aid	C. (1) No purpose that can be helped by an aid C. (2) Patient well adapted to blindness	C. (1) Merely improving where no useful purpose is served, rarely supplies motivation to use an aid. C. (2) The patient who is well adapted to blindness may be one who has made a "good thing" of his disability, is accepting all of the attentions, benefits, sympathy, etc., and feels *threatened* by any improvement in his visual status or lessening of his dependency. It is often of great importance to know who made the appointment; who brought the patient in. Is it the patient himself who is interested in a low vision examination and a low vision aid or is it a relative who has heard of this and has convinced the patient to come in for it and brought him, perhaps unwillingly?

Factor	Good Prognosis	Poor Prognosis	Comments
D. Flexibility	D. Willing to adapt to a new way of doing things	D. Inflexible	
E. Visual Field	E. Good visual field. Ability to move around	E. Insufficient visual field	E. The extent of the visual field remaining and the location of the remaining field are probably the determining factors. Thus advanced retinitis pigmentosa or advanced glaucoma lead to relatively poor prognoses.
F. Etiology	F. (1) Retinal degenerations other than retinitis pigmentosa (2) Myopia (3) Structural anomalies: albinism, aniridia, coloboma, etc. (4) Primary optic nerve atrophy (5) Diabetic retinopathy	F. (1) Retinitis pigmentosa	F. The etiology is less important than the integrity of the visual field and the extent and location of scotomas. Thus, some studies have found glaucoma a favorable condition, others have found glaucoma an unfavorable condition. Even many cases of retinitis pigmentosa and diabetic retinopathy *can* be helped.
G. Stability	G. Stable condition	G. Active deteriorating condition	G. The principal reason for the poor prognosis in diabetic retinopathy is the frequent rapid deterioration.
H. Age	H. 11 to 60 years most favorable	H. Over 80 years less favorable (many *are* helped)	H. Young children have large accommodative amplitudes and do not need to read fine print. Chronological age is not as important as mental alertness and attitudes.
I. Education and Intelligence	I. The more education, the better chance of success		I. Since the principal assistance that can be offered is for near work, the demand for near work is a determining factor. A person who is highly dedicated to reading and paper work will find a low vision aid indispensable.

Factor	Good Prognosis	Poor Prognosis	Comments
			A person with a vision loss who *never* cared to read and prefers to listen to the radio and gardening, driving and other non-close work will be less likely to need or accept a low vision aid. The extent of education may also influence the patient's ability to understand the nature of his loss and what can be done about it. Rosenbloom (1966) found even 70% of those with 1-8 years of education benefitted from aids while 81.4% of those with over 12 years of education benefitted.
J. Self-image	J. Patient has tried various magnifiers and devices on his own initiative.	J. Patient tries to conceal his vision loss and rejects any device that is odd looking or would indicate that he has a vision problem.	J. A patient, already using some device to help him utilize his vision demonstrates interest in making use of his remaining vision and shows that he does not care if people realize that he has a defect when they see the device.
K. Color vision	K. Recognizes colors	K. Defective color vision because of a large central and para-central scotoma	K. Color is important as an indicator of the extent of central vision. However, people who have no color vision because they are congenitally color blind may be very good low vision patients.

Screening Patients

Home Screening

A. Inquiry (adapted from William Feinbloom [1960].)

   1. Can the patient count another person's fingers at two to three feet?

   2. Can the patient get around in the street visually?

   3. Can the patient recognize colors? In crossing streets does he watch the lights or other people?

   4. Does the patient have a purpose for using his vision that can be met with a low vision aid?

If the answers to the above are "yes" and a specific purpose is mentioned, the patient should be encouraged to have a low vision examination even if extensive travel is involved. A negative answer on color recognition is not, necessarily, decisive.

B. Acuity Test (after John Neill [1953])

    1. 150 ft. Snellen "E" is sent with instructions for its use at 5 ft.

Neill found he had 90% success with those who achieved this acuity (5/150).

Office Screening

A. Any acuity up to 20/1000 or 20/2000 should warrant considering a low vision examination.

B. The most important screening criteria in the office is a negative one! Ignore unfavorable results found with the ophthalmoscope or bio-microscope! Too many patients have been denied the benefits of low vision aids because a practitioner skilled in the use of an ophthalmoscope was positive that no one could see very much with *that* fundus or media.

C. The home inquiry, listed in above, also can be conducted in the office.

Chapter 3

Psychological and Sociological Factors

In collaboration with HELEN M. MEHR, Ph.D.

General

Even though it has become almost a cliche among specialists that they must adopt a holistic approach, this concept is easy to forget when dealing with a patient who apparently has a specific problem such as low vision. It must not be forgotten that the eyes and vision are a part of a person. The individual's attitudes, experiences, expectations, physical and mental capabilities shape the ways in which he uses his vision and his vision affects his attitudes, experiences, expectations, etc. We cannot consider the patient or his vision alone, but we must think of the interrelationships with family, peers, employers, teachers, etc. The optometrist must consider the broad aspects of human behavior embodied in psychology and sociology.

Freud looked within the individual for the motivations of his behavior. Sullivan (1953) describes psychiatry as the study of interpersonal relationships. Haley (1963), among others, considers the extended family and gives many examples in which misinterpretation could easily be made as to the etiology of an individual's difficulties if the significant people in his life and their needs are not considered.

Working with low vision patients must frequently be regarded as part of a rehabilitation process. As such, the economic implications for the patient in terms of jobs, pensions, etc. must be considered. The effect of visual performance on dependency relationships and family role have to be kept in mind. While the immediate situation must be dealt with, the patient's long range adjustment to his disability is even more important, and everything we say, do, and recommend must have that consideration in mind.

Optometry and ophthalmology should not feel that they have the total responsibility for the social and psychological adjustment of their low vision patients. While the low vision practitioner needs to be aware of all factors affecting the rehabilitation of his patients, he often needs to involve experts from the fields of psychology, psychiatry, social work and rehabilitation.

Practitioner's Set

Influences

There is reciprocal interaction between the optometrist and his patient and the patient's family. The optometrist's psychological set is influenced by his education, his colleagues and his experiences with patients.

Attitudes

Too often in the past, the optometrist's psychological set in dealing with low vision patients has been characterized by the following attitudes:

A. Personal feelings about the patient

Before working with the handicapped, any practitioner or therapist needs to examine his own feelings and motivations. How does the optometrist feel about the visually limited? Does low vision make the patient:

1. less than a whole person?
2. Valuable to the practitioner's ego since the patient's dependency can feed the practitioner's feelings of omnipotence?
3. an object of pity?

B. Feelings about low vision care

1. "Nothing more can be done."

The patient has been referred for medical or surgical care: *"That is all I can do"*, rationalizes the optometrist. Medical and surgical care is of no further avail: *"There is nothing more to do"*, rationalizes the ophthalmologist. Simmons (1966) reports two-thirds of the ophthalmologists he studied had poor to negative attitudes toward rehabilitation.

2. "The patients reject the aids anyway."

Although repeated studies have shown about seventy percent of patients use their aids, the failure to successfully fit thirty percent seems enormous by contrast with the tiny failure ratio of routine refractive care. One or two failures may sensitize the optometrist and cause him to avoid all low vision aids in the future.

This success ratio of seventy percent is high compared with most surgical, medical and psychiatric therapies; more so, since most low vision care involves geriatric patients. The practitioner has to readjust his expectations, as well as his techniques, when he undertakes low vision rehabilitation.

3. "Fitting telescopic spectacles is both difficult and expensive."

In the Rosenbloom (1966) and Industrial Home for the Blind (1957) studies, only about ten percent of the devices used were telescopic. By contrast, over two-thirds of the devices used by the Industrial Home for the Blind (1957) were those which could be considered *ordinary* spectacles.

Fitting telescopic spectacles *is* difficult and expensive, but it is unfortunate that the field of low vision care should be considered synonymous with one of its smaller areas.

Patient's Set

Influences

A. The response to awareness of a vision loss may give rise to the following emotional reactions: shock, depression, anxiety, disbelief, grief, denial, anger. The sequence varies as does duration and intensity.

B. The patient's psychological set is determined by a large number of factors including the recency, severity, and suddenness of his vision loss. A severe, sudden loss may appear cataclysmic and throw the patient into a state of psychological shock.

Mehr, Mehr and Ault (1970) have pointed out that the person whose vision changes over a period of time has to make a continual series of adjustments and is faced with an uncertain future. This is a condition which is likely to produce an enormous amount of insecurity and anxiety.

In an emotional life crisis situation, the prior emotional strength, self-esteem, family attitudes and relations all become important influences determining the severity of the reaction and the ability to cope with it.

C. Shock and depression

1. Shock represents a period of protective emotional anesthesia. It is too painful to think about the present situation. The patient is numb. Even highly intelligent people may act slow, stupid and unresponsive.

2. Depression usually follows shock. It is characterized by: self-recrimination, feelings of self-pity, hopelessness, lack of self-confidence, suicidal thoughts and psycho-motor retardation.

A very good therapy is the judicious use of activities and tasks. If the patient can accomplish some simple thing which he thinks is too difficult, it will help in overcoming his depression. Ellerbrock (1960) suggests navigating to the bathroom alone or reading a letter with an optical aid. Cholden (1958) cautions against an overly ambitious task, since failure may intensify the depression. Raising and then shattering hope may reinduce the shock.

The family may have a critical role in determining the length and depth of depression. The Mehrs (1969) have pointed out that the family may be overly solicitous of the patient's welfare and, by overprotecting him and attempting to do everything for him, intensify his feelings of helplessness. The patient must undergo a re-evaluation of his previous aspirations, which are probably *too high* for his present status, and his concept of his present capabilities, which are probably *too low* for his present status.

The help of a psychologist or social worker in bringing out feelings and facing the aspirations and capabilities realistically may be most helpful at this point.

D. Disbelief

Many, with a recent loss, will engage in the search for a cure. They refuse to accept the diagnosis and prognosis of their doctors. "Science, faith or medical skill must surely be able to accomplish the miracle of restoring vision", they believe. At this point, they are not ready to accept a low vision aid. They are looking only for a complete and total restoration of their former visual capabilities. They will play the game of "yes, but.....",

"*If only* I could read the newspaper!"

"Well, you can read the newspaper with the assistance of this aid."

"*Yes, but* I never hold anything that close." or

"*Yes, but* I wouldn't wear anything that looks like that."

"*Yes, but*, etc., etc., etc."

Along this route of searching for a cure, the patient may have acquired a low vision aid, possibly at high cost. Since he is not willing to accept anything less than a cure at the time, he may now have acquired the attitude that: *"I've tried low vision aids and they don't work!"*

The patient's eventual rehabilitation and eventual success are better served if he understands *and is ready to accept* the limitations of any aid *before* he orders it, rather than receiving the correct prescription prematurely.

E. Denial

This reaction to illness or disability is well known and recognized in behavior exhibited by practitioners of Christian Science. It is also manifested by terminal patients, where patient, family, friends, physician and hospital staff may be part of the huge conspiracy to ignore the obvious facts and assume that the one-in-a-million chance miracle will happen (Kubler-Ross,1969).

Weinstein and Kahn (1955) point out that people are capable of refusing to admit the absence of a limb following an amputation! It should, therefore, not surprise us that there is denial of the less obvious defects, such as hearing and vision loss.

The role of the needs of the family in determining this denial reaction are less well-recognized. The charade may be unconsciously played out for the "benefit" of someone other than the patient. An attitude of denial can also be established and internalized within the personality so that the need to deny disability may continue long after the needs of the original instigator are no longer a real factor.

Usually, the denier will not accept any low vision aid, since it would require admitting his loss of vision. Occasionally, a *simple* aid will fit into his system of rationalization—e.g., "You see, there is nothing wrong with my vision, other doctors just didn't prescribe the correct lenses for me".

The Self-Image

How I see myself may bear little relationship to *how others see me* and both of these will differ from *how I really am.*

A. Imagination

Maltz (1960) points out that our assumptions are based on *imagination, not fact.* A human being performs according to what *he believes* is true of himself and his environment. Our self-image is what *we believe* to be true of ourselves.

B. Decisions and action

The input in the "rational" decision-making process will be the characteristics and capabilities the individual *imagines* he has. The degree to which this imagination differs from the perception of others and from reality will be a major factor in determining the appropriateness of the decisions and actions taken.

Thus, the person who does not have a self-image of himself as a person with a visual disability may turn away rather than admit that he did not recognize someone, or refuse to wear any conspicuous aid. Those who have a self-image of a partially - sighted person may strongly reject any aids symbolic of total blindness, such as a white cane.

C. Symbolism

The usefulness of an aid may be less significant than its symbolic meaning to the person, or what he *believes* its symbolic meaning will be to others. Likewise, the symbol of an achievement may have more influence on the self-image, or the image others form than the achievement itself. The symbolism of trophies, diplomas and degrees, in this regard, is well recognized. A self-educated man is no less well educated for lacking a diploma, but he and others fail to recognize the fact. A driver's license is symbolic proof to many people of the adequacy of their vision.

1. The aid as a symbol

Mehr, Mehr, and Ault (1970) point out that the partially-sighted, in their discussion group, were most willing to accept aids like lamps, felt pens and wide-lined paper; less willing to accept conspicuous optical aids; most reluctant to accept aids like Braille or white canes, associated with the totally blind.

2. The achievement as a symbol

Reading, to many, is symbolic of being sighted. Thus, an aid that permits reading may change a self-image from "blind" to "sighted".

To a person who has not really accepted the blind label, this may be a great morale boost. On the other hand, a person whose financial and emotional security has been oriented to a self-image of himself as a blind person may be so threatened by a low vision aid, that it is totally rejected.

Holding a certain job or driving an automobile may be so identified with vision that when the partially-sighted person achieves them, he may drop his self-image of a person with a handicap.

D. Changing the self-image

   1. Gradual erosion

Readjustment may take place with time. Thousands of incidents accumulate that are incompatible with an unrealistic self-image. Slowly, the opinions of others make an impression. Finally, the reorganization takes place, triggered by some emotional experience, possibly a movie, some overheard remark or a dream.

2. Psychotherapy

Individual or group psychotherapy may speed the process of change, forcing the person to look at himself more realistically and exposing the roots of his attitudes.

3. Hypnosis

Hypnosis offers a quick way of communicating with the unconscious. Maltz' (1960) system of psychocybernetics is, essentially, a do-it-yourself approach to changing the self-image by self-hypnosis.

4. Symbols

The value of the symbol depends on its personal import to the individual and his emotional reaction to it.

   a. Achievement with symbolic importance to the individual, e.g., reading the newspaper.

   b. External validation. Examples are:

      i. Licenses or diplomas

      ii. Jobs

      iii. Legal acknowledgement of change of status—accepting "blind aid".

      iv. The messages signalled by authority figures. Examples are: Being able (or unable) to read a chart in a doctor's office, or the pronouncement of a renowned specialist.

   c. Use of symbolic aids

It is unlikely that a strongly symbolic aid (e.g., a white cane) will be used until a compatible self-image exists. However, each time the device is used and its necessity and usefulness acknowledged, the self-image is reinforced and solidified.

5. Expectations

The individual's acceptance of his capabilities is influenced by the positive and negative expectations he feels others hold for him. Doctors, relatives, friends and other partially-sighted people may have great influence in this respect. A low vision clinic or a professionally led discussion group of partially-sighted people can be a means of positively influencing the self-image by the expectations they have for the partially-sighted.

6. Positive reinforcement

"Rewards" received for actions based on the self-image will tend to strengthen it and make it more acceptable to the individual. Examples are:

    a. Financial benefits—from Blind Aid, etc.

    b. Increased independence

    c. Increased privacy

    d. Praise

    e. Acceptance (especially where rejection and pity were expected).

A discussion group of partially-sighted people can be very useful in *d* and *e* above.

Motivation

The motivations of the patient are the important factors and should not be confused with the different motivations of relatives, social workers, rehabilitation counselors, or optometrists.

A. The too well adapted

1. Acceptance of the status of a blind person is facilitated if receipt of "blind aid" or a veteran's pension, etc. is a primary motivation. If the partially-sighted person feels that using his vision endangers these financial benefits, he will be motivated not to use it.

    a. This negative motivation may be disguised or even denied and requires great skill, clinical intuition, and outside help to diagnose.

    b. It is sometimes possible to counter this fear of using vision by pointing out that the legal and disability status will not be changed by use of low vision aids.

2. "Wooden Leg"

Dependence may be achieving more for the person than independence. Mehr and Mehr (1969) have cited the example of the grandmother with poor vision whose grandchildren spend time with her daily, reading the newspaper to her. An ability to read by herself might deprive her of the company of her teenage granddaughter (who would probably much rather be listening to a phonograph record or talking on the telephone with her friends). Berne (1964) describes this as the "game" of "Wooden Leg". The payoff is dependency; the thesis: "What do you expect of a man with a wooden leg?", or just as easily, "What do you expect of a person who is half blind?".

When the appointment is made by someone else, and some other member of the family is much more eager to have the patient helped than the patient is to receive assistance, the optometrist may well suspect a "Wooden Leg" situation.

B. Independence

The desire to cope with life, with the minimum amount of assistance from others, is a strongly positive motivation for accepting a low vision aid. The manner in which a low vision aid will help achieve this independence should be pointed out, where this is a factor. The desire to work and support self and family may be sufficient to overcome many other negative factors.

C. Privacy

Reading one's own mail or taking care of one's own financial affairs may represent a strong motivation to use low vision aids. This is especially true of adults not living with a member of their immediate family.

The Success-Oriented Examination

Rationale

With the set of other practitioners in the eye care field and the patient's set in mind, the examination provides an opportunity for the skillful low vision practitioner to promote positive attitudes in the patient. As an authority figure and an expert, the messages he gives the patient (intentionally or not) may be of greater importance than the prescription he writes.

The message that needs to be conveyed, in most instances, is "You have useable vision and I am here to assist you in using it to greater advantage".

Procedure (See Chapter VII - The Low Vision Examination)

A. Stay within the patient's capabilities.

Use large letter charts at shorter distances, working from the easily seen to the more difficult, *not* vice versa. With the 700 ft. letter of the Feinbloom Chart as a starting point, it is possible to begin testing at 5/700 or 10/700.

B. Praise his achievements.

For best results, this praise must be immediate and enthusiastic. A quick "right", "good", "excellent", or "wonderful" will get across a message that will encourage better and better performance.

C. Use tests that convey a positive message.

1. When form vision exists, use a chart to measure it, not devices like finger counting—which conveys the message "Your vision is so poor you cannot even see the chart".

2. Take the first acuity measurement after retinoscopy, using the lens you believe will produce the best acuity. To start by testing unassisted visual acuity on an aphake or high myope is to reinforce the idea that his vision is hopeless. Similarly, before a near point card is presented to the patient, calculations should be made to assure that the letters are large enough and the lens adequate to achieve reading most of the card.

3. Use charts that permit reading of a number of optotypes before the threshold is reached; 20/200 can be measured by using a chart on which only a single 200 foot letter is read, or with the Feinbloom chart used at ten feet, where the patient could achieve the reading of twelve letter sizes and twenty-four characters before stopping with the 100 foot digit. The measured acuity is the same, but the message received by the patient is much different.

4. The texts of reading cards should convey some positive messages or, at least, not painful ones, such as "taking good care of the only pair of eyes you'll ever have".

D. Use positive language.

Preferred	Poor
Low Vision	Sub-normal vision
Partially-sighted	Partially-blind
Aid	Correction
Can see	Can't see
Able	Unable
Change	Deterioration or degeneration
Unusual	Abnormal

E. Be realistic and truthful.

A positive emphasis does not imply that the patient should be told he can do things of which he is incapable. A "hard sell" approach is a prelude to future disappointment.

F. Preparing for acceptance of aids

1. The patient should understand the benefits but also the limitations of the aids recommended.

2. To insure against later rejection, the patient should know the appearance of the aid before it is ordered.

3. The patient should experience success in the office during training. Taking home an aid (without training in its use), to struggle with and use improperly, is likely to lead to frustration, disappointment and rejection.

Life Cycle Problems

There seems to be a greater incidence of adjustment difficulties of the partially-sighted as compared to the totally blind, according to Cowen et al. (1961). Blasch and Apple (1966) have noted that the partially-sighted person has a "...built-in ambiguity that makes it difficult for him to acquire a realistic self-concept. He will usually cling tenaciously to his identity as a sighted person."

Mehr, Mehr and Ault (1970) describe the partially-sighted as "the man in limbo". Unable to fit completely the role of a sighted person or a totally blind person (and, certainly, not fitting society's stereotypes of the blind), he feels misunderstood and unsure of what society and others expect of him or how they will react to him. Most partially-sighted people who acquire the condition in later life do not know others with a similar handicap. Consequently, they feel isolated and do not realize that their problems are shared by many other people (see Figure III-1).

Infants And Young Children

In the case of a young child, it is often the parents who exhibit shock, depression and, often, guilt and anxiety, as Lairy (1969) has pointed out. It is a well-accepted principle in the mental health field that an atmosphere of tension, guilt and emotional disturbance surrounding a child is bound to be undesirable for his personality development. The emotional stability, as well as understanding and intelligent handling of a handicapped youngster by parents and others, is very important in determining his future emotional strength and stability.

The young child may be made over-dependent or over-independent, according to the way in which he is treated by his parents. The optometrist can assist by realistically informing the parents of what they can expect of the youngster. Diagnostic interpretations are not enough. Specific indications and instructions regarding illumination, etc. are most helpful.

The School Age Child

It is important that the developing child be given opportunities to associate with both the sighted and the partially-sighted. The child may feel inadequate and frustrated. He may miss visual communications cues and must have substitutes in verbal and tactual form. It is important that teachers understand the size print, illumination, contrast, position relative to the blackboard, etc., information which the low vision specialist can provide. Many partially-sighted youngsters will fatigue rapidly and require extra rest periods. It is, likewise, important that their classmates be familiarized with the use and reason for any unusual low vision aids, so that the youngster will not be embarrassed in their use.

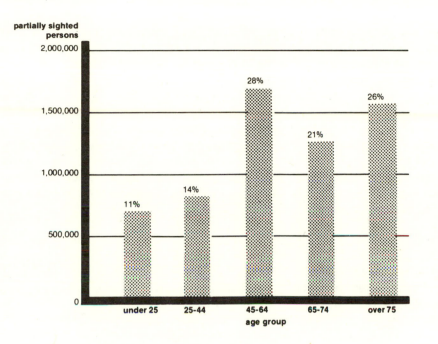

Fig. III-1. *Estimated number of partially-sighted persons in various age groups (Goldish and Marx, 1973). It is apparent that 75% of the partially-sighted population are over the age of 45 years and that 47% are over the age of 65 years. Most of those in these older age groups had an adventitious loss. Note that if the graph were to show only prevalence as a function of age there would be a sharp rise in the curve with increasing age. The figure above shows a peak in the 45 to 64 years age group since both prevalence and the size of the age groups within the population are reflected.*
Reproduced by permission of The New Outlook For The Blind.

The Adolescent

If early development is adequate, adolescence need not be *much* more difficult for the partially-sighted than the fully-sighted. Adolescence *is* a difficult time of life for *most* children in any case. Most adolescents go through a period of critical self-awareness. Real or imagined faults and disabilities are dwelt upon and magnified. An obvious disability like low vision, strabismus, nystagmus, etc. becomes a focus for self-devaluation. A visual disability does not have to result in maladjustment, assuming that the visually disabled person has constructive environmental experiences. (Cowen et al.,1961).

In dealing with adolescents, it is better to point out the consequences of behavior and let them make the decision, with limits set only for matters of safety. Lecturing or forcing is detrimental to constructive behavior. It is important for the professional in vision care not to bypass teenagers—to work directly with them, not with their parents. One has to win the youngster's confidence and guard against being put in the position of defending the parents against the child's needs and desires. Young people are usually more susceptible to the opinions of their peers than the wishes of adults.

Young people are often resistant to being different. Boys, especially, want to drive cars and seek independence. The car is often a masculine symbol or a symbol of being in control of power. Both girls and boys, at this age, are apt to be very sensitive to being different and may reject unusual low vision aids, or even ordinary spectacles.

Young Adults

Because of the emphasis in our society on physical fitness and work, the period of young adulthood is a particularly trying time for the handicapped. Individuals who cannot drive a car find the problem of transportation becoming intertwined with the problems of the emergence of independence versus the need for dependence. Consequently, the self-concept of the young adult is likely to contain many negative aspects. Usually, partially-sighted persons are not likely to have another partially-sighted person serve as a model.

The spouse and family of the young adult need to know, in detail, the abilities and inabilities of the visually handicapped person. Partially-sighted individuals and their families have a fear of injury, worsening of the disability, doubts as to their capability in the future, and doubts about a correct diagnosis. They fear embarrassment from outstanding mistakes, such as bumping someone with hot food, snubbing people, etc.

Adults

Loss of vision usually brings with it a decreased level of social status (Glass, 1970). Both with young adults and adults, the problems of employment and marriage are crucial. With recent visual loss, there is need for immediate help.

Visual loss may be symbolic to the person of a loss of sexual potency and may result in changes of the equilibrium and interrelationships between the partially-sighted individual and his family. With the change in the continuum of dependency-independency, marriages may dissolve, and the expert in vision may need to involve others in the mental health professions.

There are some visual losses that are associated with progressive deterioration due to genetically based diseases, e.g. retinitis pigmentosa. The problem of a possible transmission of visual defects through offspring creates many anxieties, and reliable help from professionals is not usually offered.

Frank discussions of the possibilities for employment and the assistance of rehabilitation agencies can help to allay fears that the partially-sighted person has that he will be totally useless. This, in turn, can prevent the deep depression that many suffer.

The Aging

Many elderly people have mixed motivations with regard to rehabilitation. Some of them would prefer to be more dependent. As in other categories, work with families is needed, and lurking fears of deterioration, etc. need to be dealt with by direct confrontation.

Varying degrees of hearing loss are common in the older population which, combined with a vision loss, may effectively isolate the individual from family, friends, and public communication media. Other senile changes such as memory loss, malfunctioning of the cognitive processes, along with decreased mobility, further complicate the maintenance of normal social relationships and communications. The demise of family and close friends or the geographical transfer to an area remote from accustomed people and surroundings further intensifies the isolation and loneliness. Any acceptable sensory aid such as a low vision or hearing aid may decrease the isolation and feelings of loneliness. Where an optical aid is infeasible or unacceptable, non-optical aids (e.g. talking books) and social services (e.g. Friendly Visitors) should be recommended.

The geriatric low vision patient can be the real test of the techniques of the optometrist. The slow reactions of the low vision patient combined with the slowed reactions of the aged require a slowed pace, extra patience, and understanding. Although the slowed pace requires additional time, visits should not be too prolonged since these same people generally fatigue rapidly.

The rehabilitation of the elderly partially-sighted person is complicated by their tendency to exhibit increased rigidity and inflexible habits. The patient's inflexibility must be met with a greater flexibility by the optometrist, who must have a diverse armamentarium of solutions.

Although the authors have discussed some of the many problems encountered with the elderly, it should also be noted that some of their favorite patients and most rewarding experiences have come from this age group. It must be emphasized that chronological age may be a misleading indicator of senility. There are "old" sixties and "young" nineties.

Communication

The impact of vision loss on written communication is so obvious that it is often overestimated. The fact that aural communication also suffers from vision loss is less well recognized. The role of non-verbal communication is not fully appreciated by the general public.

Hearing

While folklore has spread the idea that loss of vision is compensated by increased acuity of hearing, those suffering an adventitious loss of vision complain of *increased difficulty* in hearing following their vision loss. This observation of apparent hearing loss is so widespread that it cannot be ascribed to a coincidental vision and hearing loss. The apparent hearing loss is the result of missing visual clues which clarify partly audible spoken communication, e.g., a head nod or shoulder shrug may communicate a message very clearly, even if the voice is barely audible.

Feelings

The emotional content of a communication is often expressed non-verbally by body contact (e.g., a "warm embrace" or a "friendly handshake") or by visually observed body language. This visually observed non-verbal communication may be the smile that says that "you son-of-a-gun" is a friendly greeting, or the stern look, that says the same words are to be taken as an insult.

All sighted sensitive people are consciously or unconsciously attentive to facial expressions and body movements of those to whom they are talking or listening. For this reason many people will take long journeys rather than try to conclude delicate negotiations by telephone. To a large extent those with vision loss are in the position of listening on the telephone while their fully-sighted partner is enjoying many of the advantages of being physically present.

Openness
The fully-sighted learn that others read their facial expressions because they are aware that they do it themselves. Keeping a "poker face" is a socially desirable trait in our society. We must not give too visible evidence of amusement at someone else's "faux-pas". The congenitally visually impaired are apt to show their feelings more freely, not realizing that their unspoken message is being read *loud and clear*. They have to be taught this social grace, since it probably will not be acquired naturally.

Eye Contact
The importance of eye contact is recognized in many cliches and by most writers. The stereotype of the honest man is one who looks you "straight in the eye". The person ashamed will not look at you. The crook is often described as "shifty-eyed".

Not only are messages of love transmitted by eye contact, but attention is directed and gained by the same method. We obtain the attention of a person we wish to address by looking straight at him. We signify our desire not to speak by looking away.

Under these generally accepted rules of eye contact, the person with a loss of vision may be seriously handicapped. Where is the waitress or salesclerk? Is someone looking directly at him? He may see the face but not the eyes. The eccentric viewer may have great difficulty, since in order to see another person, he must not look directly at him. The sighted individual will interpret the position of the eyes as indicating an interest in someone or something else.

The lack of eye contact in communication with the visually impaired often leads to vague feelings of discomfort by the sighted participants.

Improving Communication
Those working with the partially-sighted need to be aware of the problems involved in the impairment of non-verbal communication. The professional in this field must review his own gestures, facial expressions, etc. with an awareness that the messages are lost to the person with low vision. Verbal or tactual messages can be substituted once this awareness becomes a habit.

Families, friends, employers, teachers, and the partially-sighted themselves, need to be made aware of this problem since many never realize the amount of visual communication they are using or that it is not being received in large part. This educative function of the low vision specialist is more often ignored than practiced, but it can be a very important service to the partially-sighted person and his extended family.

Chapter 4

Physiological Optics of the Abnormal Eye

General

Traditionally, the subject to be discussed in this chapter is referred to as physiological optics. In understanding low vision, we must account for not only the normal, but also the abnormal; for optics influenced by physiology *and* by pathology.

By accounting for the abnormalities and understanding their consequences, we can make reasonable predictions of the type of care or aids required.

The Cornea

Irregular or Scarred Surfaces
A. An aspheric or scarred cornea may produce irregular astigmatism or other refractive distortions.
B. Contact lenses may be the best solution to providing a new and regular refractive surface. They are extremely effective for keratoconus.
C. Pinholes and stenopeic slits are often helpful in limiting the refractive region used. Artificial pupil contact lenses have been used successfully for this purpose (Rosenbloom, 1969). Proper fitting is difficult and their use limited.
D. When the opacities become luminous sources through scattering, etc., illumination controls are indicated.

The Iris and Pupil

Hypopigmentation
A. Transparency of the iris (along with decreased pigmentation of the sclera, choroid and retina) in albinism causes light fogging and photophobia. This is usually accompanied by nystagmus and squinting of the lids.
B. Light control is indicated.

Aniridia and Coloboma
A. Excess light is transmitted.
B. Peripheral corneal and peripheral lenticular as well as extra-lenticular areas are involved in image formation causing a degradation of the image on the retina.
C. Artificial pupils and illumination controls should be considered.

Miotic Pupils
A. Age has a direct influence on pupil size and changes in pupil size. With age, the size of the pupil under conditions of high illumination decreases. But even more significantly, the amount that it can dilate under conditions of low illumination is even more drastically reduced. The graph (Figure IV-1) illustrates this change. A sixty-year-old compared to a 20-year-old experiences 1/3 the change in pupil area with change from day to night lighting and an 80-year-old 1/10 the change of the 20 year old.
B. Whether natural or drug induced (as in glaucoma) miosis requires increased illumination.

The Crystalline Lens

Cataracts
A. Opacities of the lens cause similar problems to those of the cornea. Their interference in the visual process depends on their anterior-posterior location and their position relative to the pupillary area, as well as their density.
   1. Posterior polar cataracts, because of their location near the nodal point, are especially detrimental.
   2. A central cataract may be much more of an impediment with a small pupil. Not only is illumination control required, but occasionally the near reflex, reducing the pupil size, may cause such a problem that the use of relative distance magnification is impractical. If other factors are favorable to its use, a mydriatic may be indicated.
   3. Because of nuclear sclerosing, with its accompanying color distortion, and because fluorescence of the lens from ultra-violet results in a haze, the eye with cataract generally prefers incandescent light to fluorescent. It is also in need of protection from bright sunlight.

Subluxation
A. If a condition of double refraction exists, it may be controllable by pinholes, stenopeic slits or pupil contact lenses.
B. When an artificial aperture is contemplated, the refraction should be done with it in place.

Aphakia
A. All the usual problems of fixed focus, increased magnification (an asset to the low vision patient), field limitations, aniseikonia, anisophoria, strong lenses, spatial disorientation and increased transmission of ultra-violet are present.
B. Bifocals in ultra-violet absorbing glass or plastic are required. Unfortunately, one sees aphakes, especially children, with low acuities, wearing only distance corrections. A *high* add, rather than no add, is required.

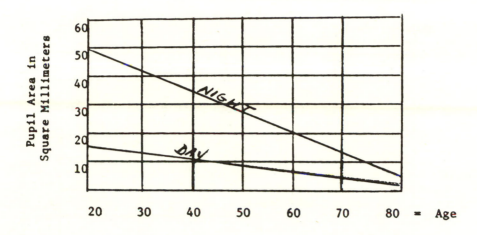

Fig. IV-1.   Pupil size as a function of age (Keller, 1971). Reprinted by permission of the Journal of the American Optometric Association.

The Vitreous

Floaters

A. Floaters in the vitreous constitute a variable impediment to vision.

B. Large floaters may be shifted by eye movements so as to reduce their occlusion of the visual axis.

C. If eye movement causes annoying intrusion of floaters, movement of the object may be substituted for eye movement.

The Retina, Optic Nerve and Visual Pathways

The Retina

The dual organization of the retina with rods and cones and their different characteristics and distribution become important when some of these structures do not function normally.

A. Deficient rod function (as in retinitis pigmentosa) results in night blindness or decreased rate of dark adaptation and loss of peripheral vision.

B. Deficient cone function (as in macular degeneration) results in changes in visual acuity which are dependent on the retinal area involved, changes in color vision, and in extreme cases, loss of day or photopic vision.

C. When visual acuity is plotted as a function of retinal locus (Figure IV-2), the concentration of cones and their greater neuron supply in the macular area result in the characteristic spiked curve with visual acuities dropping off rapidly for para and peri-macular areas. However, damage in a retinal region need not result in total loss of function. In many degenerative diseases an increase in illumination may produce results as startling as magnification.

D. The phenomenon of contour interaction has been described by Flom, Weymouth and Kahneman (1963).

This effect increases as the para-macular areas are used for vision. Consequently, it is characteristic of persons with central scotomas to miss central letters on eyecharts and to have

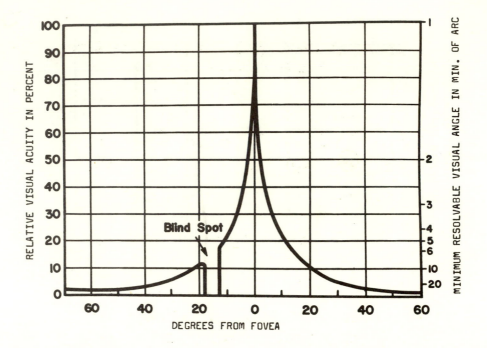

Fig. IV-2.   *Visual acuity as a function of retinal locus (Gregg and Heath, 1964). Copyright 1964 by D. C. Heath and Company. Reprinted by permission of the publisher.*

greater difficulty with larger words in reading. The near point number chart, designed by Feinbloom (Figure IV-3) is very good for indicating the difficulty that contour interaction will cause. With an intact macula and minimal contour interaction, the patient will read the multiple digits if he can read the single digits. With greater amounts of contour interaction, there will be greater difficulty in reading double digits and still more for multiple digits, even though isolated single digits of the same or sometimes smaller size are readily recognized.

E. Ability to recognize colors demonstrates the presence of functioning cones.

Some pathological processes are selective in the retinal elements affected. Tritan color defects rarely occur on a hereditary basis but commonly occur with diseases of the outer (receptor) layers of the retina. Acquired red-green defects are more commonly associated with affections of the conductive layers of the retina and of the optic nerve (Kollner, 1912).

Many low vision patients, who can recognize colors, are unable to perform on pseudo-isochromatic plate tests. The Farnsworth Dichotomous Test Panel D-15 (Figure IV-4) is easily and rapidly administered and can be used with low vision patients by allowing them to get closer and take more time than normal.

If the spectral sensitivity of a patient can be determined, it may then be possible to prescribe a color filter for optimum visual enhancement.

Scotomas And Field Defects

There has been a great tendency to predict success or failure of low vision care on the basis of etiology. However, the characteristics of the remaining visual field, *whatever the etiology*, will determine the potential for success.

NEAR READING CARD FOR PARTIALLY BLIND
Arranged by WILLIAM FEINBLOOM, Ph.D.
for: DESIGNS FOR VISION, INC.

24 Point

7 2 6 5 8 3 1 4 9

25 47 89 63 71 35

18 Point   **Children's Books**

6 9 3 4 1 5 8 2 7

22   43   87   91   40   16

14 Point   **Books**

4 8 6 5 7 1 3 0 2

21   48   63   75   92   87

385   726   491   832   647

10 Point   **Text Books**

1 5 8 3 9 2 0 7 6

59   86   49   71   36   29

831   479   136   508   268

7 Point   **Newspaper**

3 8 2 7 6 4 1 5 8

50 93 76 81 24 22

284 175 906 382

5 Point   **Newspaper**

7 4 3 5 1 6 2 9 8 5 7

90 74 83 62 58 47

971 358 9016 482

4 Point   **Small Bible**

1 4 2 7 6 5 8 3 2 7 4

82 14 79 46 56 23

7206 565 4831 579

Copyrighted

Fig. IV-3. *Feinbloom near point number chart. Reprinted by permission of Designs For Visions, Inc.*

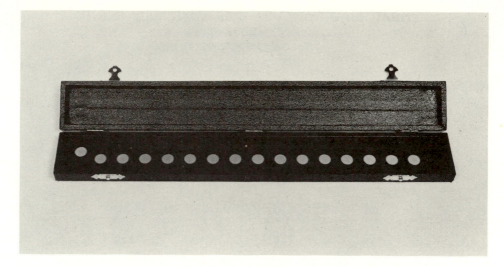

Fig. IV-4. Farnsworth Dichotomous Test Panel D-15. The test consists of a series of 16 colored papers which the subject arranges in order of closest hue match. The arrangement, selected by the subject, when plotted on the analysis sheet indicates the status of color vision, and the type of defect if abnormal. This test easily indicates the colors that a color deficient subject will confuse.

The location, extent and density of scotomas and field restrictions will be a major factor in determining the ease and extent of visual performance.

A. Central Scotoma

This always causes decreased visual acuity. If the surrounding para-macular tissue is healthy and intact (as in macular cysts), magnification around the central defect works very well.

B. If the macula is surrounded by other damaged tissue (as in some macular degenerations), or the scotoma is more extensive (as in optic atrophy), eccentric viewing as well as magnification may be required.

C. The proximity of a scotoma to a favored viewing area may decrease its usefulness. In Figure IV-5, the scotoma to the right of the macular area would be very disabling to a person reading a language read from left to right since the next word would always disappear.

Possible solutions to this problem are turning the page upside down and reading from right to left or turning the page 90 degrees and reading vertically.

A scotoma immediately to the left of the macular area will cause problems in finding the beginning of a line of print. Use of the finger as a marker can overcome this problem.

D. Large field defects such as hemianopsias cause mobility problems. These are more severe if the defect encompasses the inferior field of both eyes. Mobility training is indicated for these conditions.

E. Concentric field restrictions which result in a small remaining central field (as in retinitis pigmentosa or glaucoma) cause problems in mobility and in locating objects in the surround. If reasonably good visual acuity remains, a reverse telescope can be used to create a minified image of a larger area on the useable retina.

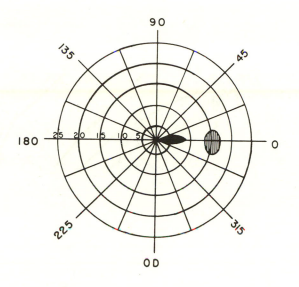

*Fig. IV-5.   Tangent screen plot of a scotoma located imme-
diately to the right of the fixation point.*

Fixation

A. Eccentric fixation

Occasionally an eccentrically fixating, and consequently amblyopic, eye remains as the more useful one after loss of vision to the normally fixing eye. In this situation, pleoptics may offer the best chance of restoring centric fixation and better acuity.

B. Eccentric viewing

More frequently in low vision care the problem is one of learning to use a para-macular area for seeing when the macula is no longer functional. If this occurs later in life, a well developed system of fixation based on the macular area already exists. Even though the patient uses a para-macular area for years, he always realizes that he is not looking directly at the object. This type of eccentric viewing means a continual effort to look away from the central region and can be quite fatiguing. Sometimes it is better to magnify the image to extend around the central scotoma, if this will produce sufficient acuity, since the fixation problems will be simplified (see Figure IV-6).

C. Nystagmus

With congenital losses of central vision (as in albinism), nystagmus is usually present. The nystagmus is almost always a result of the poor vision—not its cause. Nystagmus from congenital vision loss does not cause the patient to see the world in motion.

Although nystagmus is not a detriment to the use of low vision aids, further improvements in acuity may be realized if the rate or extent of eye movements is reduced. For a particular patient, those factors which affect the nystagmus should be investigated. e.g., direction of gaze, illumination, nervous tension, fatigue, uncorrected refractive error, etc.

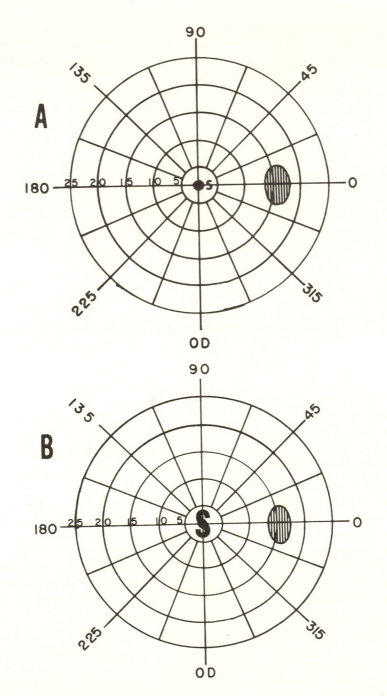

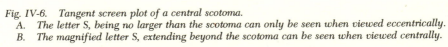

Fig. IV-6.   Tangent screen plot of a central scotoma.
   A.   The letter S, being no larger than the scotoma can only be seen when viewed eccentrically.
   B.   The magnified letter S, extending beyond the scotoma can be seen when viewed centrally.

Magnification may decrease the nystagmoid movements and thus increase acuity more than the amount of magnification would indicate. Where nystagmus is primary, the increased angular magnification may magnify the effect of the oscillations causing little visual improvement or even a decrease in visual acuity (Rosenberg and Werner, 1969).

Lateral nystagmoid movements increase contour interaction problems in the horizontal meridian. Turning a page 45 degrees or even 90 degrees can improve the spacing in the horizontal meridian and thus improve discrimination of letters or numbers in a line of print.

Chapter 5

Magnification

General

Magnification may be defined as "an increase in the apparent size, the perceived size, or the actual size of an object, or of its image in relation to the object" (Schapero et al., 1968). The purpose of magnification, regardless of the method of obtaining it, is to increase the size of the retinal image. The size of the retinal image may be specified in terms of the angle subtended at the center of the eye's exit pupil. This angle is proportional to the angle subtended by the object at the center of the eye's entrance pupil. Thus, the larger the angular subtense of the object *as seen by* the eye, the larger the angular subtense of the retinal image. Therefore, methods of magnification increase the angular subtense of the object *as seen by* the eye.

For purposes of low vision management there are basically four ways in which the angular subtense of the object at the eye may be increased. They are:

1. Relative size magnification
2. Angular magnification
3. Relative distance magnification
4. Projection magnification

Total magnification in a given instance may result from a combination of these types. Such combinations are especially effective since the total magnification is the *product* rather than the sum of the individual types.

E.g. Relative Size Magnification   =   3×
Relative Distance Magnification   =   5×
Total Magnification   = 15×

Relative Size Magnification

Definition

Relative size magnification is that magnification brought about by increasing the actual size of the true object. This can be done with many kinds of objects, perhaps the most familiar being large print. Other examples are: large eyed needles, large T. V. screens, enlarged photos, etc.

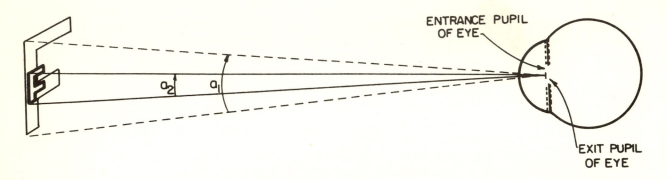

Fig. V-1. *Relative size magnification.*

Formula

Since it is the object subtense at the eye which is important, the magnification is expressed in terms of the tangent of the angles subtended by the objects at the eye (See Figure V-1).

$$M_S = \frac{\text{Tan } a_1}{\text{Tan } a_2}$$

M_S = Relative size magnification
a_1 = Angular size of enlarged object
a_2 = Angular size of initial object

Obviously, it is not necessary to specify an object distance as long as it is the *same* for both objects.

Type Notations

A. Point type

For teachers and librarians, the customary standard for the initial object is 10 point. A point is 1/72 of an inch in height. However, the measurement is made on the type slug rather than the letter. Actual size of the printed letter is dependent on type style, upper or lower case, letter, ink spread as well as point size.

For optometric purposes it is necessary to keep in mind that the relative point size designations are only *approximately* related to the actual magnification, e.g., 12 point print is *only* approximately twice the size of 6 point print. See Table of Type Equivalents. (Figure V-2).

B. Jaeger

The Jaeger system is *totally* hopeless for predicting magnification from the designations. While higher Jaeger numbers represent larger print than lower Jaeger numbers, there is no consistent relationship between number designation and change in print size.

C. M Notation

The M system (meter letter size for Snellen notation) gives exact results. Thus, a 3M letter is exactly three times the size of the same 1M letter, just as a 60 foot letter on a distance Snellen chart is three times the size of a 20 foot letter. This system has the additional advantage that the test distance can be measured in the same unit (meters) and a Snellen fraction written. Snellen's basic formula is:

$$V = \frac{d}{D}$$

V = visual acuity
d = test distance
D = distance at which test letter subtends 5 minutes

E.g., A 2M letter read at a test distance of 10 centimeters (0.10 meters) can be written 0.10/2.00 and readily compared to its equivalents 10/200 or 20/400.

D. Equivalent Snellen

"Equivalent" Snellen notations (e.g. 20/40 equivalent at 16 inches) give exact results for magnification since a 20/40 letter is twice the size of a 20/20 letter. However, the system is confusing since the numerator does not indicate the actual test distance and is cumbersome if the test distance is varied from the one specified. Fortunately, most optometric near point charts have been designated for use at 40 centimeters. This makes conversion to M notation a matter of simple mental arithmetic. By multiplying the denominator of the "equivalent" letter size by 0.02 it becomes the M letter size, e.g., 20/50 equivalent at 40 centimeters becomes 1.0M.

Type Legibility

A. Legibility of type is not only dependent upon size, but also upon the configuration of the type. Figure V-3 shows the results of a study of type faces versus legibility by Prince (1965).

B. Prince outlined the following characteristics of large print to improve legibility for the visually handicapped:

1. The print should have clean edges.

2. The print should be of such a size that the lower case "o" will approximate 2.7 mm. or more in the vertical direction. The strokes should not be too bold—not more than 17.5 percent of the letter height. These dimensions favor 18 point type.

3. The paper should have high contrast and good opacity. It should also be light in weight.

4. The line length should not be less than 36 picas.

5. Periods and commas should, if possible, be larger than those traditionally used. The period should be approximately 30 percent of the lower case "o", the comma should be approximately 55 percent of the height of the lower case "o".

6. Hyphenation should be kept to a minimum, preferably eliminated entirely.

Merits of Large Print

A. Disadvantages

1. Availability

Few books are available in large print and the attempt to print a large selection would be prohibitive. Even if feasible it would be an inefficient expenditure of time and money because almost anyone who can read large print can read ordinary print using other methods of magnification.

TEST TYPE EQUIVALENTS

Height of Letter (mm.) (1)	Jaeger Test Types (2)	Point Type Lower Case (3)	Digits Points (4)	M (5)	20/20 Equiv. @ 40 cm.	Point Type Upper Case (6)	Uses (7)
0.6	1	3		0.4	20/20		
0.8	2	4		0.55	20/23		Mail Order Catalogs
0.95	3	5		0.65	20/33		Classified Ads
1.1	4		4	0.75	20/38		
1.2	5	6		0.85	20/42	4	Classified Ads, Footnotes
1.45	6	8	5	1.00	20/50		Telephone Directory
1.6	7	9		1.10	20/55	6	Magazines, Textbooks
1.75	8	10		1.20	20/60		Newspapers, Magazines, Textbooks
1.9	10	12	7	1.30	20/65	8	Elite Typewriter, Children's Books (Grades 4-7)
2.3	11	14	10	1.60	20/80	9	Children's Books (Grades 1-3)
3.1	12	18	14	2.15	20/108	12	Children's Books (Pre-School), Large Type
4.0	14		18	2.75	20/138	14	
4.4		24		3.00	20/150	18	Large Type Books
5.1	16	30	24	3.50	20/175		Display Advertising
8.4	18			5.75	20/287	36	
10.8	19			7.40	20/370		
17.0	20			11.65	20/583		

1.   Height of Letters: For M size and 20/20 equivalents, interpolations can be made.

2.   Jaeger types vary. These measurements are based on B & L Card 713568-101, and Dr. Ziegler's which are in reasonable agreement with each other. The letters measured were lower case "e" and "o".

3.   Measurements (averaged) on samples of lower case "e" and "o" mainly taken from "A Manual of Style", by University of Chicago Press.

4.   Sizes of digits vary. There are lower case and upper case digits. These measurements were made on Near Reading Card for Partially Blind, arranged by William Feinbloom.

5.   M sizes are the calculated distance in meters at which a letter height (first column) subtends a 5' angle.

6.   Measurements averaged on samples of upper case type. The letter measured was usually "T".

7.   Examples of usage are based on lower case point type size.

Fig. V-2. Table of type equivalents. Measurements were made by the authors using a magnifying comparator of the type generally used for measuring contact lenses. Tables of type equivalents vary with the particular samples used and should only be considered as approximations for other samples of type. For accuracy and consistency, it is recommended that the letter height of a sample be measured and converted to the type notation desired using this table.

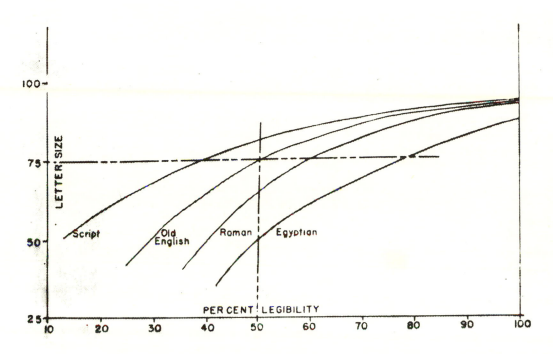

Fig. V-3. *Legibility curves of four different type faces from the study by Prince (1965). Note that sans serif Egyptian face can be smaller size than the other three faces and still be more legible. Reprinted from Book Production Industry; December, 1965 by permission of the publisher.*

2. Book size (see Figure XV-1)
Large print obviously results in both larger and thicker books and papers. In most cases, it is nearly impossible to hand carry large print novel length editions. Furthermore, many single volume works become multiple volumes when converted to large type, thus, creating difficulties when referring to other sections of the work.
3. Because of the simplicity of the large print approach, some partially-sighted patients may resist learning to use other types of magnifying devices after becoming accustomed to large print. *Early* exposure and training with magnifying aids would increase the independence of the patient and the scope of materials available.

B. Advantages
1. Large print books permit unrestricted fields of view and allow more normal working distances than most optical aids.

2. Large print is advantageous in beginning reading training of the visually handicapped, where it is better to have as few complicating factors as possible. Large print also serves well in early stages of training with low vision aids.

Angular Magnification

Angular magnification is the ratio of the angle of subtense of the image formed by an *optical instrument* compared to the angle of subtense of the actual object. Thus, angular magnification is the ratio of the *apparent* size of the object as seen through the instrument compared to the *true* size of the object. The classic example is the magnification produced by a telescope.

All types of magnification *can be* specified in terms of angular subtense. However, less confusion results when the term "angular magnification" is reserved for instances where magnification does *not* result from *changes* in *object size* or *object distance*.

Relative Distance Magnification

Definition

Relative distance magnification is that magnification which results from reducing the distance between the object and the eye. From Figure V-4, it can be seen that angular subtense is increased by this method.

Formula

$$M_d = \frac{x}{x'}$$

M_d = Relative distance magnification
x = Comparison distance
x' = New distance

Magnification resulting from distance changes is inversely proportional to the two distances, e.g. if the target distance is decreased to one-third, the angular subtense is tripled resulting in 3X magnification.

Microscopic Systems

A. Although some "angular" magnification may be induced by microscopic spectacle systems, relative distance magnification is by far the most important factor. Simply stated, the purpose of high plus spectacles for near magnification is to allow the patient who otherwise has insufficient accommodative facility to focus the object clearly, at a very short distance.

B. As the object and lens are moved away from the eye, relative distance magnification decreases. However, angular magnification increases until it eventually becomes the more important factor. The total magnification, which is the product of relative distance and angular, is constant (see Figure V-5).

C. When relative distance magnification is induced without the use of a visual aid such as in the case of high myopes or youngsters with adequate accommodative facility (see Figure V-6), there is no artificial limit placed on the field of view. Thus, many of *these* patients will not accept a low vision aid unless performance improvement is marked. Also most low vision patients prefer to move one-half as far (M=2X) from the TV set rather than utilize a 2X telescopic which restricts the field of view.

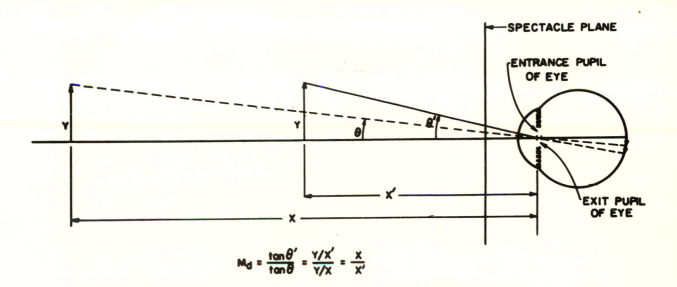

$$M_d = \frac{\tan\theta'}{\tan\theta} = \frac{Y/X'}{Y/X} = \frac{X}{X'}$$

Fig. V-4.   *Relative distance magnification.*

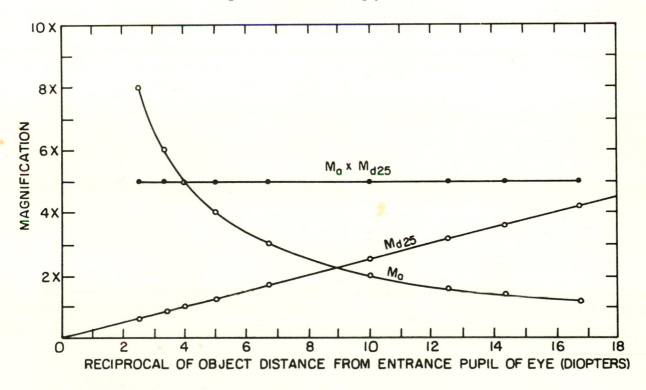

Fig. V-5.   *Angular (M_a), relative distance (M_d), and total ($M_a M_d$) magnification plotted for a +20.00 D. lens with the object in the primary focal plane of the lens. The reference distance for relative distance magnification was taken as 25cm. Note that the total magnification is the same as the effective magnification referred to 25cm. ($M_{v25} = F/4$)*

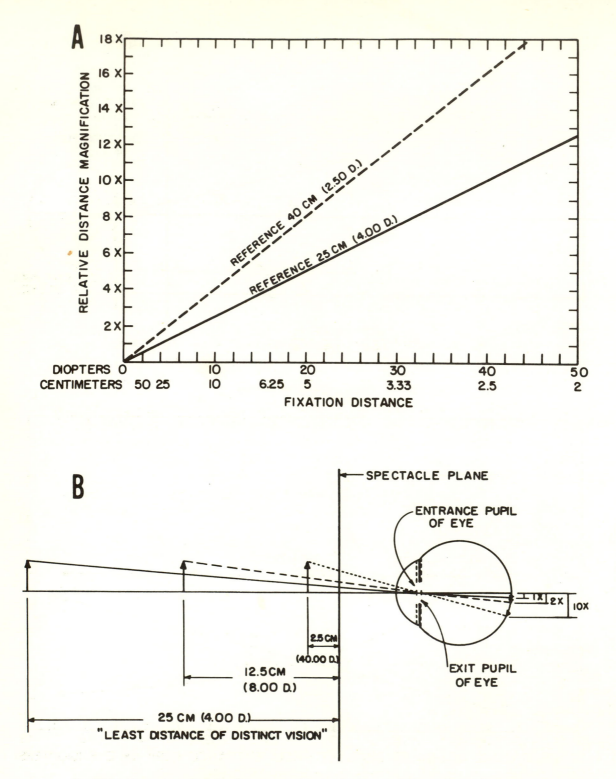

Fig. V-6A. Comparison of relative distance magnification for 40cm. and 25cm. reference distances.
  B. Drawing showing increased retinal image size resulting from decreased object distance. Note that linear object size remains constant while angular size increases.

D. Figure V-6 demonstrates the relative distance magnification for different fixation distances as compared to a standard fixation distance of 25 cm., ("least distance of distinct vision").

Projection Magnification

Definition
Projection magnification may be defined as that magnification which results when an enlarged image of an opaque or transparent object is produced on a screen.

Optical Projection
Until recently, projection magnification always involved some form of optical projection device. These consist of a light source, an optical system and a screen. Compact opaque projectors with translucent screens have been designed for the partially-sighted (see Figure V-7).

Electronic Projection
Recently, several groups, Potts et al.(1959), Genensky et al.(1968), Weed et al.(1968), Lavieri and Wilson (1972), and others have devised closed circuit television magnification systems (see Figure V-8).

Devices based on the work by Genensky et al. at Rand have been marketed. The basic magnification obtained with these systems is produced electronically rather than optically. One may vary the electronic magnification by changing the monitor size or vary optical magnification by changing the lens system of the television camera.

A. Major advantages of electronic over the optical projection magnifiers are:
1. the provision of increased "working space" by divorcing it from working (viewing) distance, thus allowing customary eye to object distances and space for manipulation of pencils, needles, tools, etc.;
2. ability to increase or decrease image brightness (purely optical systems are all "light losers");
3. capability of increasing contrast;
4. control of background illumination ("glare") by changing black on white to white on black.

B. Major advantages of electronic magnifiers over optical aids (spectacle or hand held) were found by Mehr et al. (1973) to be:
1. possibility of contrast reversal
2. contrast enhancement
3. increased depth of focus because of greater working distance
4. binocularity with large amounts of magnification because of greater working distance
5. reduction of aberrations and distortion
6. reduction of postural tension
7. reduction of necessity for saccadic movements, beneficial for those with very narrow fields or using eccentric viewing
8. significantly increased duration of reading time
9. ability to read smaller print by contrast enhancement and feasibility of greater magnification
10. some increase in reading speed
11. improvement in ability to write and perform other hand-eye tasks because of increased working space.

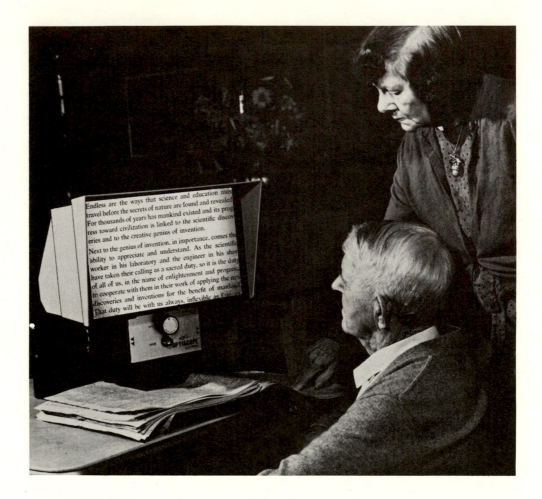

Fig. V-7.   *The Optiscope, an optical projection magnifier. Photo courtesy of Opaque Systems Ltd.*

C. Many improvements can be incorporated into electronic systems if cost limitations can be overcome:

    1. contrast enhancement by control of "grey scale"
    2. automatic focusing
    3. zoom optics
    4. multiple cameras
    5. multiple monitors
    6. split screens
    7. recording and playback
    8. miniaturization
    9. etc., etc.

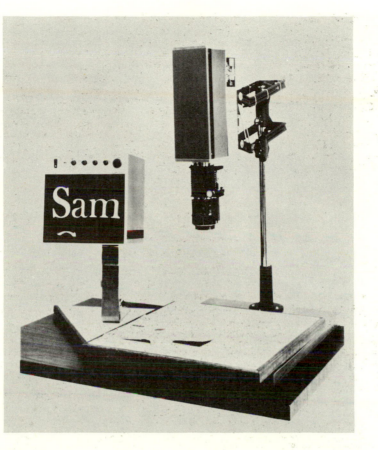

Fig. V-8.   *An early model of a closed circuit television magnification system. Photo courtesy of Apollo Lasers, Inc.*

Total Magnification

As with relative size magnification, the amount of magnification produced by a projection magnifier itself, is independent of the viewing distance. However, the total magnification afforded to the patient is the product of that magnification by projection and that magnification produced by the decreased viewing distance (relative distance magnification). Thus high orders of magnification are possible without the limitations of field and distortions imposed by strong optical aids.

Disadvantages

The most serious disadvantage to all projection magnifiers is the cumbersomeness of the equipment. In addition, the optical projection magnifiers are limited in the form and location of material which can be magnified. Another factor limiting their use has been their relatively high cost.

Chapter 6

Optics

Microscopes, Loupes, and Magnifiers

General

All of the systems to be discussed under this category are basically convergent systems which allow viewing of objects at short distances from the lens system (no more than the focal length). The complexity of various systems is related to efforts to reduce aberrations thereby increasing the useable clear vision field.

A. Although these systems do afford "angular magnification", this is a minor consideration relative to the magnification due to the proximity factor if the lens is close to the eye (seeFigure VI-1) and is usually ignored in microscopic spectacles (see Chapter 5 Magnification, Relative Distance Magnification). A more accurate estimate of the total magnification results from the product of the angular magnification and the relative distance magnification.

B. High power lenses suffer greatly from various optical aberrations resulting in serious restrictions on the size of the useable field as well as deterioration in the quality of the image. Thus the higher power systems require aspheric surfaces, and/or multiple lens combinations, and/or reduced lens diameters, in order to minimize these effects. Most low vision practitioners begin to consider the use of more sophisticated systems for lenses of +12.00 D. and above.

Assumptions

A. In utilizing these systems the object is placed at or a small distance within the primary focal point. This results in an enlarged erect image with the image distance always greater than the object distance.

B. By manipulating the object to lens and/or lens to eye distance, the image is positioned within the accommodative facility of the patient.

C. The resulting magnification is a function of the image distance from the eye (see Figure VI-2).

D. To compare magnification of different systems, an arbitrary standard viewing distance must be established. This is usually 25 cm. (the traditional "least distance of distinct vision"). Sloan and Habel (1957) and Brazelton (1969) have recommended the use of 40 cm.

E. Southall (1933a) defines the magnifying power of a convergent optical system used in

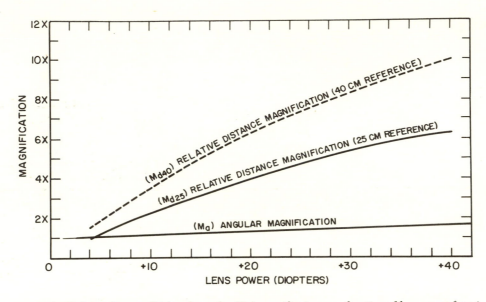

Fig. VI-1.   *Relative distance (M_d) and angular (M_a) magnification as a function of lens power for microscopic spectacles. Calculations assumed: "thin" lenses; magnification at the eye's entrance pupil, 1.7cm. behind the spectacle plane; object located in primary focal plane of lens; and reference distances of 25 and 40cm. measured from the spectacle plane.*

conjunction with the eye as the ratio of the apparent size of the image as seen through the instrument to the apparent size of the object as it would appear at the "distance of distinct vision" (25 cm.).

Magnification Formulae
The magnification specified for a particular system depends upon the magnification formula used. The formulae vary in terms of reference point, whether objects or images are being compared, and how the particular system is used (accommodation).

A. Angular magnification
   1. This is the magnification induced by the lens system itself, without regard to relative distance magnification.
   2. Angular magnification compares the angular image size (formed by the magnifier) to the angular object size.

$$M_a = \frac{\tan \theta'}{\tan \theta}$$

M_a = angular magnification
θ' = angular size of image
θ = angular size of object

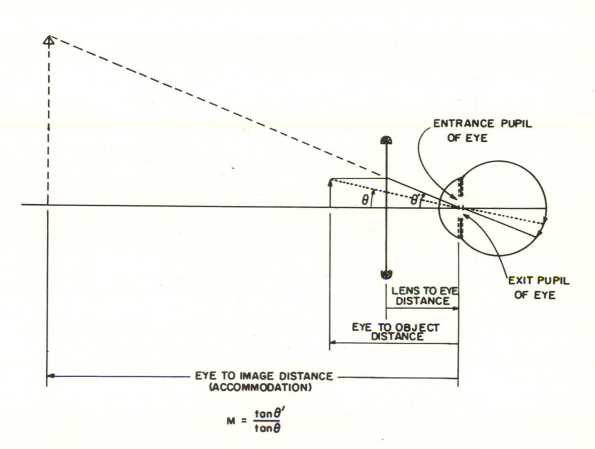

Fig. VI-2. *Magnification with a convex lens.* θ *is the angle subtended by the object at the eye's entrance pupil.* θ' *is the angle subtended by the image at the eye's entrance pupil.*

3. If the object is in the primary focal plane of the lens:

$$M_a = 1 + hF$$

M_a = angular magnification
h = distance from the lens to the eye's entrance pupil (meters)
F = lens power

Figure VI-3 shows the relationship of the various elements of this formula.

4. If $h = 0$ in the above formula, as is the case if the lens were at the entrance pupil of the eye, M_a becomes unity. As the lens is moved away from the eye the angular magnification increases.

5. It is important here to realize that this situation does *not* result in increasing retinal image size. Because the object is in the primary focal plane of the lens the retinal image size remains *constant*, regardless of the lens to eye distance. However, the apparent (angular) size of the *object* decreases as the system is removed from the eye and thus the comparison of sizes results in an increased angular magnification.

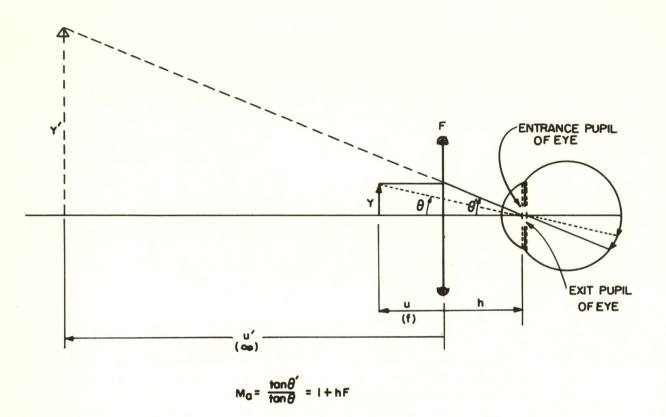

$$M_a = \frac{\tan\theta'}{\tan\theta} = 1 + hF$$

Fig. VI-3. Angular magnification (M_a) with the object in the primary focal plane of a convex lens.

6. When a lens (and object) is near the eye, angular magnification is minimal and relative distance magnification the more important factor. As the lens (and object) recede from the eye, angular magnification increases while relative distance magnification decreases. The total magnification remains constant. Hence, for a presbyopic emmetrope, the same strength needed in a spectacle lens to resolve print can be used in a hand magnifier at arm's length (see Figure V-5).

B. Relative distance magnification with spectacle lenses

1. Probably the most commonly used magnification formulae relate to relative distance magnification.

2. The following formula specifies the magnifying power of an optical instrument with the eye as a reference point (the most stable reference point for a specific eye is its entrance pupil):

$$M = d\ [F-A\ (1-hF)]$$

d = reference distance in meters (always positive in sign)
F = power of optical system
A = vergence of the image rays entering the eye
h = distance from lens to eye in meters (positive sign)

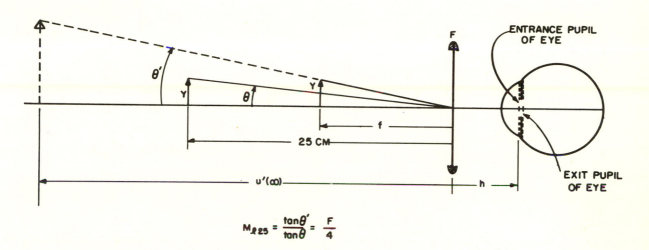

$$M_{\ell 25} = \frac{\tan\theta'}{\tan\theta} = \frac{F}{4}$$

Fig. VI-4.   *Effective magnification referred to 25cm. (M$_{e25}$). Note, despite the optical illusion in the drawing, the linear sizes of Y at the primary focal point and Y at 25cm. are equal.*

The derivation of this formula involves assumptions. First, the eye is stationary resulting in only a small portion of the field being *sharply* imaged on the retina, thus allowing the use of paraxial ray formulae. (If the eye moves, the visual angle must be related to the center of rotation, and the apparent size of the image will depend upon the angular rotation.) Second, the assumption is made that the eye is relaxed relative to accommodation.

3. If the object is at the primary focal point of the lens, the image becomes infinitely distant and A becomes zero.

Thus:

$$M_e = dF \qquad\qquad \text{EFFECTIVE MAGNIFICATION}$$

Further, if the reference distance is taken as ¼ meter (25 cm., the traditional standard), then:

$$M_{e\,25} = \frac{F}{4}$$

if the reference distance is taken as 40 cm., then:

$$M_{e\,40} = \frac{F}{2.5}$$

The "F/4" formula compares the apparent size of an infinitely distance image of the object formed by the optical system to the apparent size of the object if it were at 25 cm. from the system. Thus a comparison is made between an image requiring no accommodation and an object requiring 4.00 D. of accommodation (see Figure VI-4). This formula assumes that all refractive error has been corrected other than by the lens power under consideration and that no accommodation is in use when viewing the object through the lens.

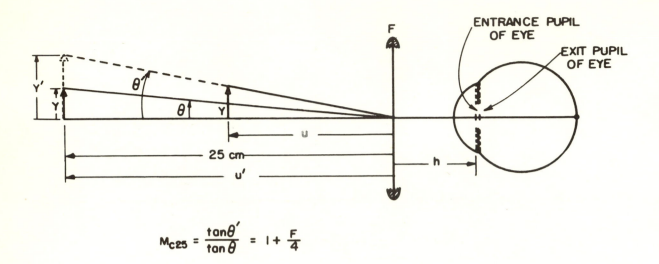

$$M_{c25} = \frac{\tan\theta'}{\tan\theta} = 1 + \frac{F}{4}$$

Fig. VI-5. Conventional magnification referred to 25cm. (M_{c25}). Note, despite the optical illusion in the drawing, the linear sizes of Y at the object distance u and $\bar{Y}$ at 25cm. (distance d) are equal.

If all ametropia has *not* been corrected then the formula becomes:

$$M_e = \frac{F - A}{4}$$

where A is positive for hypermetropia and negative for myopia.

4. Some feel that it is more realistic to compare an image distance requiring the same accommodation as the standard object distance (see Figure VI-5). In this case, A becomes -1/d.

$$M_c = d \left[F - \left(\frac{-1}{d} \right)(1 - hF) \right]$$

The distance, h, is usually small in comparison to d and thus is commonly neglected, resulting in:

$$M_c = 1 + dF$$

If d again is taken as 25 cm., the formula then becomes:

$$M_{c\,25} = 1 + \frac{F}{4} \qquad\qquad \text{CONVENTIONAL MAGNIFICATION}$$

This formula compares the apparent size of the image formed at 25 cm. from the eye by an optical system to the apparent size of the object if it were at 25 cm. from the eye. This formula also assumes that all refractive error has been corrected by means other than the lens power under consideration, and that 4.00 D. of accommodation is utilized with and without the lens.

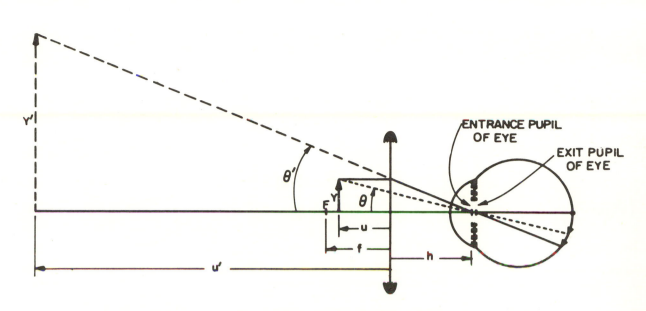

Fig. VI-6. *Angular magnification* (M_a) *where the object is within the focal distance of a convex lens.*

5. Despite appearances, these two formulae are not in conflict, but rather represent the same principle under different conditions. The "Effective Magnification" formula, $M_{e25} = F/4$, compares the apparent size of an infinitely distance image to the apparent object size at 25 cm. while the "Conventional Magnification" formula, $M_{C25} = 1 + F/4$, compares the apparent size of the image formed at 25 cm. to the apparent size of the object at 25 cm. Thus in the second formula the extra unit of magnification is produced by the 4.00 D. of accommodation required to view the image clearly at the 25 cm. distance.

C. Magnification where the object is within the focal distance

The previously discussed formulae for angular and effective magnification are based on the assumption that the object is in the primary focal plane of the lens. This assumption is not always met in practice, especially in the cases of hand-held magnifiers and some stand magnifiers. Unfortunately, many manufacturers specify the magnification of loupes and stand magnifiers based on the effective or conventional magnification formulae. It is less confusing and more accurate to specify them in terms of dioptric power, diameter, and object distance if fixed.

When the object is located between the primary focal plane and the lens, an enlarged, virtual, erect image results thus affording magnification. The formulae for quantifying the magnification in these instances become somewhat cumbersome.

1. Angular magnification

If distances measured in the direction of the light rays are positive and distances measured opposite to the direction of the light rays are negative (see Figure VI-6) then:

$$M_a = \frac{u - h}{u - h \, (1 + Fu)}$$

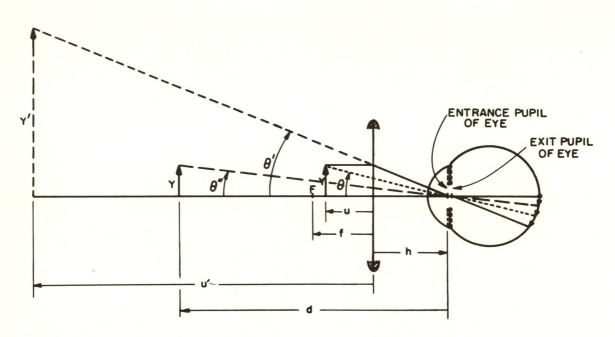

Fig. VI-7. Angular magnification (M$_a$) where the object is within the focal distance of a convex lens, compared to a standard object distance (d).

where:

Ma = Angular Magnification
u = Object's distance from the lens (meters)
h = Distance from lens to the eye (meters)
F = Power of the lens (diopters)

(In the case of thick lenses, the distances are measured from the principle planes of the lens.)

2. Angular magnification compared to a standard object distance
  a. If one wishes to compare the angular size of the image at any distance to the angular size of the object viewed without the lens if it were at a standard distance (d) (see Figure VI-7)

$$M_{ad} = \frac{d}{u - h\,(1 + Fu)}$$

b. Customarily d is specified as the "least distance of distinct vision", 0.25 meters.

Then:
$$M_{a25} = \frac{-0.25}{u\text{--}h\,(1+Fu)}$$

or

$$M_{a25} = \frac{-1}{4\,[u\text{--}h\,(1+Fu)\,]}$$

c. If the object is in the primary focal plane of the lens u = f and M_{a25} = F/4 which, as previously discussed is called effective magnification.

D. Summary of Magnification Formulae

Type of Magnification	Definition	Formulae	Assumptions
1. Angular	Compares apparent size of image formed by lens system to apparent size of object viewed without lens system	$M_a = \dfrac{u\text{-}h}{u\text{-}h\,(1+Fu)}$ $M_a = 1 + hF$	Object distance less than primary focal distance of lens system Object is in primary focal plane of lens system (u = f)
2. Compared to a standard object distance	Compares apparent size of image formed by the lens system to the apparent size of the object if it were located at some arbitrary distance. Traditionally this object distance has been specified as 25 cm.	$M_{a25} = \dfrac{-1}{4[w\text{-}h\,(1+Fu)]}$ $M_{e25} = \dfrac{F}{4}$ (Effective magnification) $M_{c25} = 1 + \dfrac{F}{4}$ (Conventional magnification)	Object distance less than primary focal distance of lens system Object is in primary focal plane of lens system 4.00 D. of accommodation required to view the image clearly if the eye is emmetropic

E. Special paradoxical considerations
   1. Lens effectivity
      a. Most vision care practitioners believe that as a convex lens system is moved away from the eye, the effect is the same as substituting a stronger lens in the original lens plane. While this is true for ametropic corrections, it is not true for near adds.
      b. Asher (1970) has pointed out that for convex lenses this tenet is true for near adds only for

the situation where the object is not closer than two focal lengths from the lens. (For thick lenses measurements should be from the principle planes.) Furthermore, he has shown that for objects closer than two focal lengths, as the lens is moved away from the eye and closer to the object, the effect is to *lessen* the power effect of the lens.

c. When using convex lenses as low vision adds, where the object is within the primary focal distance, moving the lens away from the eye and closer to the object does not increase power effectiveness, but rather reduces it. Only when the ametropic correction is greater than the add, does moving the lens away from the eye result in greater plus power effect.

2. Perceived magnification

When an object is viewed through a convex lens system, as the object and the lens are moved away from the eye, the magnification *appears* to increase and the object *appears* to enlarge. This perception occurs even if the object is in the primary focal plane of a convex system where the image rays emanate parallel, thus resulting in a constant retinal image size for all lens to eye distances.

This paradox results from the subtense of the lens diameter at the eye becoming smaller as the lens recedes while the subtense of the object as imaged by the lens remains unchanged. This causes the image to fill more and more of the area of the lens. The brain, assigning a constant size to the lens diameter (a function of size constancy), resolves the paradox by concluding that the image has enlarged.

Field Of View

A. The size of the field of view of a simple microscopic lens system is dependent upon:

1. Diameter of the lens system

This parameter is subject to various interpretations depending on whether the entire lens diameter is chosen or that diameter which is useable, often called the clear field.

2. Power of the lens system

3. Location of the reference point in the eye

4. The diameter of the pupil of the eye (Westheimer [1957] states this effect is minor)

B. One may consider the field of view relative to a stationary eye or a moving eye. The field of view of a microscopic relative to a *stationary* eye might be designated as the *static* field of view, while that relative to a *moving* eye might be termed as the *dynamic* field of view. The dynamic field of view is the field of fixation through the lens.

C. Westheimer (1957) has derived the following formulae for the extent of the field of view in the object space

$$\text{linear extent} \quad Y = \frac{c\,(h-u+Fuh)}{h} \qquad \text{angular extent} \quad \tan a = \frac{c\,(h-u+Fuh)}{h\,(h-u)}$$

Y = ½ linear extent of object plane seen through the lens
a = ½ the angular extent of the field of view in the object space (positive, meters)
c = ½ the diameter of the area of the lens to be considered (positive, meters)
h = the distance from the lens to the eye's reference point in meters (positive)
u = the distance from the lens to the object in meters (negative)
F = lens power in diopters

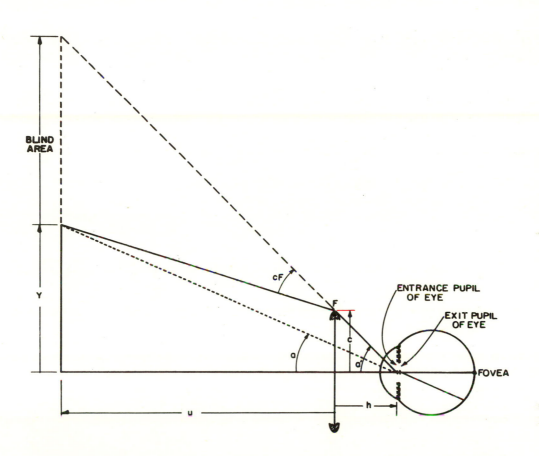

Fig. VI-8.   *Field of view for peripheral vision of a stationary eye with a simple microscope. (Westheimer, 1957).*

1. For the stationary eye (see Figure VI-8), it is assumed that:

a. The eye is stationary with the primary line of sight coincident with the optic axis of the lens.

b. The microscopic system is a thin spectacle lens. Spectacle lenses in the powers used as low vision aids are usually not "thin" and therefore some error will be introduced by this assumption. For thick lenses measurements would have to be taken relative to the entrance and exit pupils of the lens system.

c. The eye's pupil is negligibly small (see section 5 below).

d. The eye's reference point is the center of the eye's *entrance pupil*.

2. For the moving eye (see Figure VI-9), it is assumed that:

a. The microscopic is a thin spectacle lens.

b. The eye's pupil is negligibly small (see section 5 below).

c. The eye's reference point is the eye's *center of rotation* which is fixed and lies on the foveal line of sight as well as the optical axis of the lens system.

3. From the assumptions stated above and the accompanying figures, it is apparent that the real

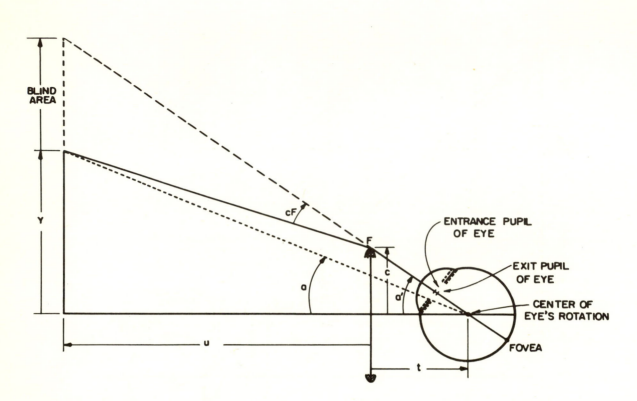

Fig. VI-9.   *Field of view for foveal vision of a moving eye with a simple microscope. (Westheimer, 1957).*

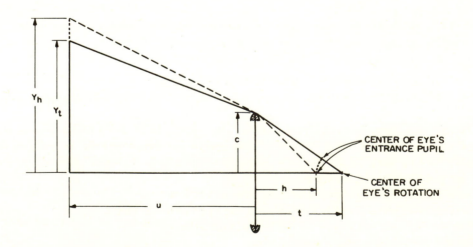

Fig. VI-10.   *Comparison of linear field of view for peripheral vision of a stationary eye and for foveal vision of a moving eye. Y_h represents ½ the field of view of the stationary eye (static field) while Y_t represents ½ the field of view of the moving eye (dynamic field). (Westheimer, 1957).*

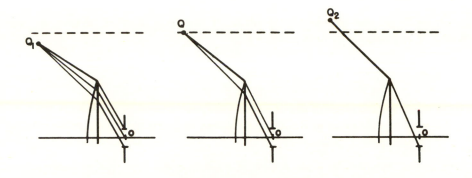

o = CENTER OF ENTRANCE PUPIL

Fig. VI-11. Effect of pupil size on the linear field of view. Rays from object point Q₁ when refracted by the lens fill the whole of the entrance pupil. Rays from Q reach the center of the entrance pupil and fill the lower half of the entrance pupil. The ray from Q₂ just grazes the bottom edge of the entrance pupil.

The range of object points from Q₁ to Q₂ will be imaged on the retina of the eye with continuously decreasing illumination. Q will be the center of the range. (Westheimer, 1957).

difference between the static and dynamic fields of view is the reference point specified in the eye. Because the center of rotation of the eye is located at a distance farther from the lens than the center of the eye's entrance pupil, it is apparent that the extent of the field of view will be larger for a stationary eye than for a moving eye, if all other parameters are the same (see Figure VI-10).

4. As Westheimer points out, if the size of the microscopic lens system is such that rays from the object reach the entrance pupil without passing through the lens, they may form retinal images of those portions of the object. These images, however, will not form a continuum with those formed by rays passing through the lens. As can be seen in Figures VI-8 and VI-9, for a convex lens system there will be a portion of the object field that will neither be imaged through the lens nor outside it. This results in a "blind area" in the object field.

5. Westheimer further discusses the effect of finite pupil sizes on the extent of the field of view. He has shown that the size of the pupil determines the range of object points whose retinal images show a gradual decreasing level of illumination (see Figure VI-11). He concludes that even a relatively large entrance pupil of the eye will not produce a significant range in view of the magnitude of the other quantities. In any case the range will be centered about the object point related to the center of the eye's entrance pupil and thus this is still the most useful measurement point.

6. Because reading aids for low vision patients are used with the object at near distances, and because the practitioner's real interest is how much reading material can be seen through the lens at any one time, Westheimer suggests the use of the linear extent formula rather than the angular extent formula.

7. If the object is in the primary focal plane of the lens (as with many spectacle plane microscopics), Westheimer's formula reduces to:

$$Y = \frac{c}{hF}$$

Y = ½ linear extent of the objective plane seen through the lens.
c = ½ the diameter of the area of the lens to be considered (positive, meters)
F = lens power in diopters.

D. As has been stated, the *useable* field of view of a microscopic lens system is dependent not on the overall diameter of the system but rather on the diameter of the area through which a clear image can be seen. This area is not easily calculated by the clinician. Hence, the authors recommend the best procedure to be followed is for the practitioner to view an object through the lens as it is to be used, and to measure the actual extent of the minimally aberrated field.

Lens Form
A. General
Because of the high powers used in low vision aids, lens aberrations become a very important limiting factor in determining the clear field of vision through a given lens. The question often arises whether low vision patients appreciate lenses that minimize aberrations. In high powers the differences are marked. In lower powers individual patients may or may not appreciate the optical improvement.
The six aberrations of lenses which must be considered are:
1. Spherical aberration
2. Coma
3. Distortion
4. Chromatic aberration
5. Marginal radial astigmatism
6. Curvature of field
There are different ways of minimizing these aberrations which may have an effect on the usefulness of a specific lens in a specific situation. Besides the power, consideration must be given to the manner in which lenses are used (e.g., the same power lens used in the spectacle plane or held 30 cm. away may require reversal of the curves used [see Figure VI-12]).
B. Controlling aberrations
1. *Spherical aberration* occurs when marginal rays passing through a lens system are brought to a focus on the axis at a point closer to the lens than the paraxial rays are focused.
Spherical aberration can be minimized by the proper selection of lens curves, reduction of the lens diameter (size or stop) or by using aspheric surfaces.
Spherical aberration is relatively ineffective as an obstacle in microscopic spectacle systems since the pupil of the eye acts as an aperture stop to limit the size of the area of the lens through which useful rays pass at any instant (Bechtold, 1953).
2. *Coma* is due to the unequal refracting effects on oblique rays of the peripheral compared to the central zones of a lens system relative to oblique light rays. Coma is spherical aberration for oblique light (Sheard, 1950).

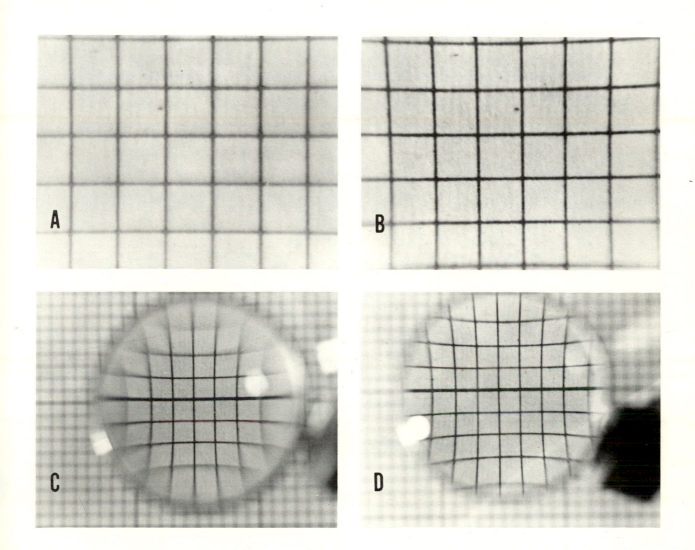

Fig. VI-12.   *Grid photographed through a 6X aspheric convex lens.*
   A.   Lens in "spectacle plane", the more convex surface toward object.
   B.   Lens in "spectacle plane", the less convex surface toward object.
   C.   Lens 30cm. in front of "spectacle plane", the more convex surface toward the object.
   D.   Lens 30cm. in front of "spectacle plane", the less convex surface toward the object. When the lens is used as a spectacle (A,B), the distortion is less when the more convex lens surface is toward the object (A). When the lens is used as a hand loupe (C,D), the distortion is less when the less convex lens surface is toward the object (D).

   The pincushion distortion is even more apparent when the grids are viewed by a human eye than for the camera. On a human retina, the image of a grid would be of equal size when the lens is in the spectacle plane or 30cm. away, provided the grid remained in the primary focal plane of the lends.

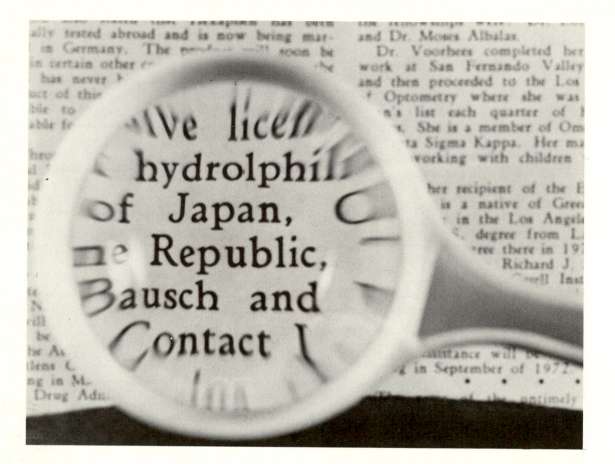

Fig. VI-13. Effect of pincushion distortion on the image of printed matter.

Coma can be minimized for a specific set of conditions by the proper selection of lens curves or limiting the lens aperture.

Like spherical aberration, coma as a blur producing obstacle is relatively unimportant because the pupil of the eye acts as an aperture stop. However, the presence of large amounts of coma has an effect on the other aberrations (e.g. astigmatism) where the distances of the microscopic lens from the eye cannot be precisely fitted and maintained (Bechtold, 1953).

3. *Distortion* is due to differences in magnification of object points away from the optical axis of a lens system. Convex lenses result in pincushion distortion (see Figure VI-13).

    a. In single lenses distortion can be reduced by using steep or aspheric base curves or limiting lens diameter.

    b. In lower powers most spectacles and other aids can be made in adequate diameters without compensation.

    c. In higher powers or large diameters aspheric curves are the method of choice.

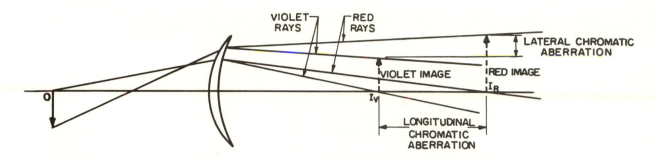

Fig. VI-14. Longitudinal and lateral chromatic aberration.

d. In multiple lens systems, distortion can be neutralized by the proper selection of individual component lens powers with an appropriately placed stop between them

4. *Chromatic aberration* involves two separate but related considerations. *Longitudinal* chromatic aberration is the variation of image distance along the optical axis with different wave lengths of light. *Lateral* chromatic aberration is the variation of image size with different wave lengths (see Figure VI-14). Correcting one type of chromatic aberration does not necessarily imply correction of the other. Lateral chromatic aberration is related to rays being dispersed by the prismatic effect of lenses. Since the prismatic effect increases the farther the rays strike from the optical axis, lateral chromatic aberration can be lessened but not eliminated by reducing the distance from the optical center that rays may strike the lens. Either type of chromatic aberration can be corrected by the use of multiple lenses having different dispersions.

5. *Marginal astigmatism* is due to light rays impinging on a refractive surface obliquely. Thus, if uncorrected, any ray striking a lens away from the optical axis will result in some degree of marginal astigmatism. The degree of astigmatism for a given lens form is dependent upon the obliqueness of the rays and the distance from the lens to the center of rotation of the eye. Hence, marginal astigmatism increases as one looks away from the optical axis and toward the periphery of a lens.

Marginal astigmatism may be minimized in single lenses by limiting the diameter of the lens or by proper selection of base curves, spheric or aspheric. In multiple lens systems it can be minimized by the proper choice of lenses to neutralize each other's effect.

6. *Curvature of field* is due to the difference in curvature between the image sphere of a lens and the conjugate focal sphere of the eye. The two spheres may be coincident on the optical axis, but the two spheres separate as the line of sight approaches the margin of the lens. This aberration may be thought of as an increasing power error as the line of sight moves from the center toward the margin of the lens.

Curvature of field can be minimized by the use of stops, steep base curves, aspheric lens forms, or multiple lens systems.

C. Interaction of aberration control

1. As lens power increases, the major interfering aberrations in microscopic systems become more of a problem. Hence, as power increases, lens diameter usually decreases.

2. In lower powers chromatic aberration is allowed to stand. Where chromatic aberration does become a factor in imagery, multiple lens systems are used.

3. For minimization of distortion, curvature of field and marginal astigmatism, proper selection of lens curves, aspheric lens curves, incorporation of stops, or multiple lens systems are used to reach the best compromise between these three monochromatic aberrations.

D. Spherical lens forms

1. Bier (1970) gives the following specifications for Lederer lenses: for a +16.00 D. lens the front curve is +20.00 D. and for a +24.00 D. lens, the front curve is +24.00 D. This design is supposed to allow a large distortion free field with adequate correction of marginal astigmatism and curvature of field.

2. An improved series of Lederer-type lenses by Stigmagna (Bier, 1970) with emphasis on correction of marginal astigmatism, and distortion held to a minimum, specifies a shallower form than the original Lederer specifications (e.g., for +12.00 D. power, the front curve is +14.75 D.; for +16.00 D. the front curve is +16.00 D.; and for +20.00 D. the front curve is +17.50 D.).

3. Fonda (1965) states that between the powers +8.00 D. and +14.00 D., lenses appear thinner when ground with a back plano surface. He further recommends for the largest useful field for a spherical lens in powers above +14.00 D. the front curve should range from +14.00 D. to +16.00 D. (e.g., a +20.00 D. lens should be ground with a front curve of +16.00 D. and a back curve of +4.00 D.). These appear to be flatter but not too different from the aforementioned forms.

4. Because it is not possible to totally eliminate marginal astigmatism in single spherical lenses above +8.00 D., and in stronger powers this aberration restricts the useable field, Bechtold (1953) recommends doublets in powers of +16.00 D. to +24.00 D., and triplets in powers of +32.00 D. to +48.00 D.

E. Nonaspheric versus aspheric form

1. Where the combination of power and lens diameter results in significant reduction in the useable field of view through the lens, one solution is the use of aspheric surfaces. For full diameter spectacle lenses, many low vision practitioners begin to consider aspheric forms at +12.00 D. and above.

2. Davis (1969) has calculated and shown field plots for different lens forms manufactured by American Optical Company. His conclusions are, for use as microscopic lenses, that there is only slight advantage to an aspheric over a nonaspheric lens for powers below +16.00 D. From +16.00 D. to +20.00 D. (the limit of the currently available series) Aolite aspheric cataract lenses do offer an advantage over their single lenses with spherical surfaces. In this range little improvement would result from a specially designed series for an object distance equal to f (Davis, 1970). In powers of +24.00 D. and above, aspheric lenses have been designed especially for use as microscopics.

3. The best decision, in any case, would result from actually trying the different forms on an individual patient to determine any differences in performance and patient preference.

F. Fresnel lenses

1. A Fresnel lens is a lens whose surface is made up of a series of stepped concentric zones, which allows powers in larger diameters without requiring the incumbent thickness of continuous surface type lenses (see Figure VI-15). The power and/or angle of the individual

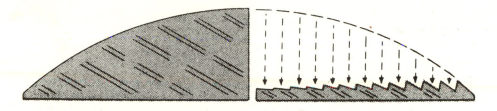

Fig. VI-15.   Cross section of a convex lens and an equivalent Fresnel lens.

zones may be varied independently thus allowing for minimization of aberrations. In recent years Fresnel lenses have also been made available in vinyl material which can be attached to a standard hard lens.

2. The advantages of Fresnel lenses are:

   a. Large diameters are possible.

   b. The thickness is minimal and uniform across the full lens diameter.

   c. They are light weight.

   d. Minimization of aberrations is accomplished easily.

   e. Large amounts of decentration are possible to control prismatic requirements.

3. The additional advantages of Press-On membrane lenses are:

   a. Convenient as temporary lens powers for training purposes, which can be changed in the office

   b. Produces availability of non-stock bifocal additions and prism segments

   c. Allows non-stock bifocal segment positioning

   d. Allows great freedom in positioning the segment's optical center

4. The disadvantages of Fresnel lenses are:

   a. The main detriment of the Fresnel lenses presently available is the loss of contrast. Many low vision patients have great problems with any reduction in contrast and reject any aid that has this effect.

   b. Patients have objected to the appearance of rings on the lenses due to the step between sections. The Press-On Fresnels have reduced the appearance of these rings, thus making this criticism minimal.

   c. When a Press-On lens is used to create a bifocal segment, the edges are more noticeable to the wearer and others than is the case with fused bifocals.

Front Versus Back Focal Length

A. When lenses are used to correct ametropia, the important consideration is that the *secondary* focal point of the lens is coincident with the far point of the eye. If the location of the *secondary* focal point relative to a physical point on the lens is to be used to designate lens power, then the *posterior* pole of the lens affords the only consistent tangible reference point regardless of lens thickness or form. Consequently, the reciprocal of this distance (*back* vertex power) has become the standard designation for ophthalmic lenses designed for ametropia corrections.

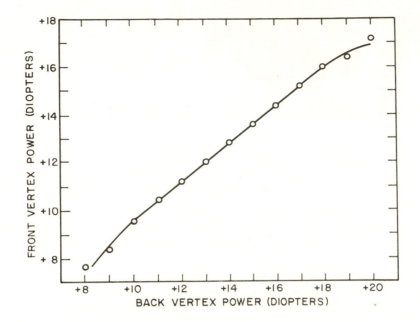

Fig. VI-16.   *Front vertex power versus back vertex power for American Optical Company plastic aspheric cataract lenses (data courtesy of John Davis, 1971). For this and other convex lens forms where the front surface curvature is greater than the back surface curvature, the front vertex power is always less than the back vertex power.*

B. When lenses are used to image a near object at a longer distance, the important considerations are the locations of the object and the *primary* focal point of the lens. In this case, the *anterior* pole of the lens affords the only consistent tangible reference point on the lens regardless of lens thickness or form. Consequently, *front focal length* is the best means of assuring consistent focal effects of test lenses and prescription lenses when used for near vision. For this reason, the powers of bifocal additions are designated in *front* vertex power.

C. One consideration, which often may be overlooked, when practitioners use cataract lenses as microscopics, is the proper designation of power. Lens powers for cataract lenses are in terms of back vertex power. Microscopics, on the other hand are designated in terms of front vertex power. In these lenses, where form and thickness may become a real factor, considerable error may result from ordering the tested microscopic power without proper compensation for the correct designation of the prescription lens. Figure VI-16 is a graph prepared from data supplied by John Davis (1971) showing the front vertex power for specified back vertex powers of aspheric cataract lenses manufactured by American Optical Company.

Telescopes

General

A. An afocal telescopic system may be defined as a lens system which results only in angular magnification (see Chapter 5, Magnification).

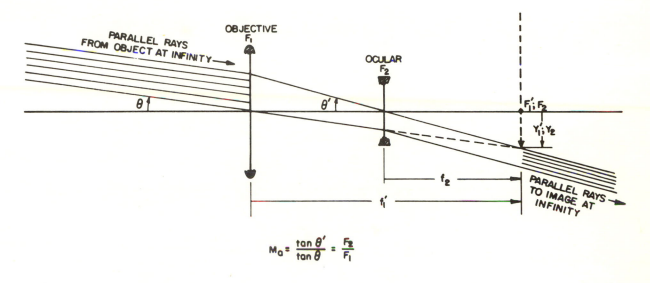

Fig. VI-17.   *Diagram of the optics of a Galilean telescope.*

B. Telescopic devices may be afocal or focused for some finite distance. Telescopic angular magnification is produced by the afocal system alone. The magnification produced by focal elements is due principally to relative distance magnification. When the effectiveness of the convex power of the objective is increased so that the telescope is focused for a near object, the device is referred to as a telemicroscope or, popularly, a telescopic loupe.

C. Telescopic systems may be regarded as a combination of *two* optical systems.

1. The *objective* (relatively large in diameter to collect a large quantity of light) is that lens system closest to the object and is a convergent system.

2. The *ocular* or eyepiece, composed of the lenses closest to the eye may be a convergent or divergent system depending upon the type of telescope. When a convergent ocular is used, an inverted image results unless an erecting system is incorporated. When a divergent ocular is used, an erect image results. A divergent ocular also results in a shorter overall device length than that which results when a convergent ocular is used. Thus to afford an erect image with minimum device length, most low vision telescopic aids utilize divergent oculars. This type of device is known as a *Galilean* telescope.

3. The objective lens of the telescope converges parallel incident rays to form a real inverted image of the object in its secondary focal plane. This image is inspected with the ocular (eyepiece) lens. When the telescope is adjusted for infinity (for use with an emmetropic eye), the secondary focal point of the objective glass is coincident with the primary focal point of the ocular glass, and hence, the entire system is afocal, resulting in emerging parallel rays (see Figure VI-17).

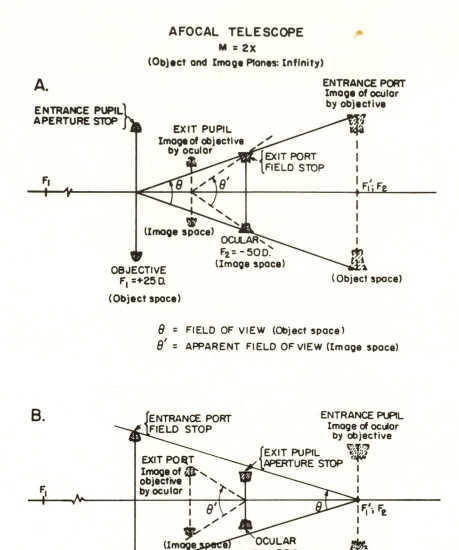

AFOCAL TELESCOPE
M = 2x
(Object and Image Planes: Infinity)

θ = FIELD OF VIEW (Object space)

θ′ = APPARENT FIELD OF VIEW (Image space)

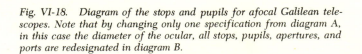

Fig. VI-18.   *Diagram of the stops and pupils for afocal Galilean telescopes. Note that by changing only one specification from diagram A, in this case the diameter of the ocular, all stops, pupils, apertures, and ports are redesignated in diagram B.*

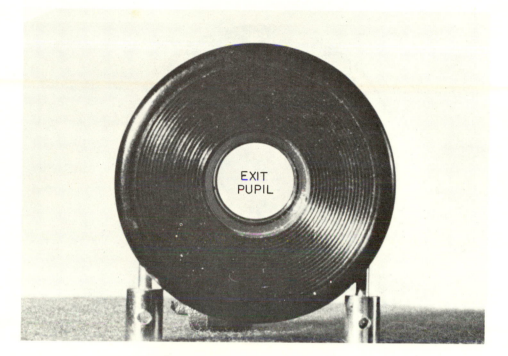

Fig. VI-19.   *Exit pupil of a Galilean telescope as viewed from image space. The exit pupil shown here is a virtual image of the objective formed by the ocular.*

Stops and Pupils

A. In determining the specific stops of a telescope, all apertures or images of apertures in the image space (i.e., those seen from the image plane) must be compared separately from those in the object space, (i.e., those seen from the object plane). Apertures or images in image space must not be compared to those in object space.

B. The real or apparent aperture, located in image space, subtending the smallest angle at the image plane is called the *exit pupil.* (see Figure VI-18).

Thus the exit pupil can be determined by viewing through the telescope from the image plane and noting the smallest real or apparent aperture (see Figure VI-19). In most cases, the exit pupil is the image of the outline of the objective lens formed by the ocular lens. In a Galilean system the above type of exit pupil is a virtual image located between the objective and ocular lenses.

C. When the exit pupil is a *real* aperture, that aperture is also the *aperture stop* (see Figure VI-18B). When the exit pupil is an *image*, then the *real aperture* in object space related to that image is the *aperture stop* (see Figure VI-18A). The aperture stop limits the size of the bundle of light rays from any object point which pass through the telescope.

D. The real or apparent aperture, located in object space, which subtends the smallest angle at the object plane is called the *entrance pupil* (see Figure VI-18).

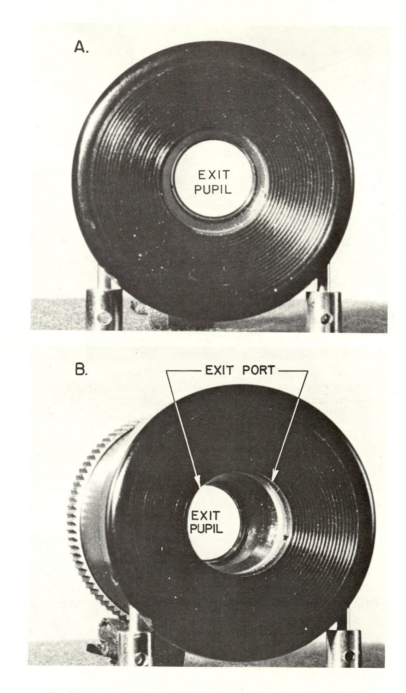

Fig. VI-20.   *Determination of the exit port of a telescope by angling the telescope.*
  A.   *Full exit pupil seen in direct view.*
  B.   *Exit pupil reduced in size by the exit port as telescope is angled.*

E. The real or apparent aperture, located in image space, which subtends the smallest angle at the center of the exit pupil is called the *exit port* (see Figure VI-18). If the exit port is a *real* aperture, that aperture is also the *field stop* (see Figure VI-18A). When the exit port is an *image*, then the *real aperture* related to that image is the *field stop* (see Figure VI-18B). The exit port of a telescope can be located by viewing through the telescope from image space, angling the telescope, and noting which real or apparent aperture in image space first reduces the exit pupil to half diameter (see Figure VI-20).

F. The real or apparent aperture, located in object space, which subtends the smallest angle at the center of the entrance pupil is called the *entrance port* (see Figure VI-18).

G. All of the above definitions are related to consideration of a telescope *alone*. Since in considering a Galilean telescope alone its exit pupil is usually between the ocular and objective and thus the eye's entrance pupil cannot be made coincident with it, and since in most telescopes the diameters of the objectives and oculars and their images are usually larger than the eye's pupil diameter, the eye's pupil becomes the limiting aperture (aperture stop) in the telescope-eye combination. Thus the specifically designated stops are different from those of the telescope alone (see Figure VI-21). In this instance the exit port is the image of the objective in the image space of the telescope-eye combination and the exit pupil is the eye's exit pupil. Thus, the apparent field of view is determined not only by the diameter of the eye ring (the image of the objective formed by the ocular [see B-2 under *Magnification* below]) but also by the distance between the eye ring and the eye. This explains why the field of view of a telescope is larger, the closer the telescope is held to the eye.

Magnification

A. In Figure VI-17 it can be seen that the magnification is: $M = \dfrac{\theta'}{\theta}$ It is further apparent that:

$$M = \frac{\tan \theta'}{\tan \theta} = \frac{\dfrac{Y}{f_2}}{\dfrac{Y'}{f_1}} = \frac{f_1}{f_2} = \frac{F_2}{F_1}$$

The positive value of M means that the final image is erect.

1. These expressions assume that the telescope is focused for infinity and that any refractive correcting lenses are added behind the ocular, thus the telescopic system, itself, may be considered as being afocal.

2. It is possible, however, to correct for spherical refractive errors or various object distances by adjusting the distance between the objective and ocular lenses.

   a. With a given object distance for hypermetropes the inter-lens distance would be longer than the afocal setting and for myopes shorter.

   b. For shorter object distances, the distance between the objective and ocular lens will be longer than the afocal setting.

   c. Varying the interlens distance is commonly used in focusing binoculars where a center post adjustment is used to set one tube for infinity and the ocular of the other tube is then adjusted to a focal match. The center post adjustment is then used to adjust both tubes for varying object distances.

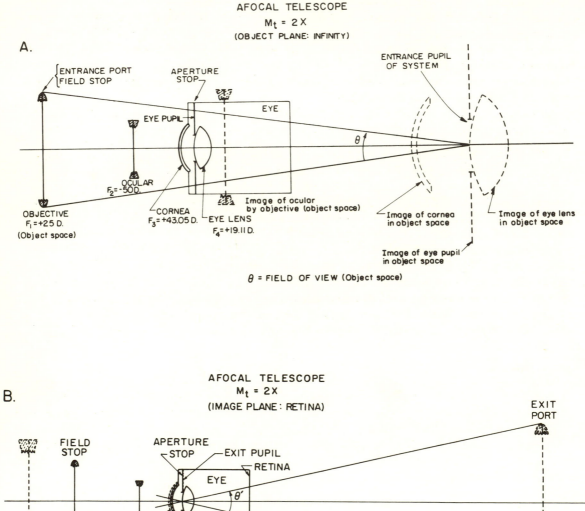

AFOCAL TELESCOPE
M_t = 2 X
(OBJECT PLANE: INFINITY)

A.

ENTRANCE PORT
FIELD STOP

APERTURE
STOP

EYE

ENTRANCE PUPIL
OF SYSTEM

EYE PUPIL

OCULAR
F_2 = -50 D.

θ

OBJECTIVE
F_1 = +25 D.
(Object space)

CORNEA
F_3 = +43.05 D.

EYE LENS
F_4 = +19.11 D.

Image of ocular
by objective (object space)

Image of cornea
in object space

Image of eye lens
in object space

Image of eye pupil
in object space

θ = FIELD OF VIEW (Object space)

AFOCAL TELESCOPE
M_t = 2 X
(IMAGE PLANE: RETINA)

B.

EXIT
PORT

FIELD
STOP

APERTURE
STOP

EXIT PUPIL

RETINA

EYE

θ'

OCULAR
F_2 = -50 D.

OBJECTIVE
F_1 = +25 D.
(object space)

EYE
PUPIL

CORNEA
F_3 = +43.05 D.

EYE LENS
F_4 = +19.11 D. (image space)

Image of eye pupil
in image space

Image of cornea
in image space

Image
of
ocular in
image
space

Image of objective
in image space

θ' = APPARENT FIELD OF VIEW (image space)

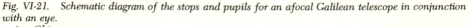

Fig. VI-21. *Schematic diagram of the stops and pupils for an afocal Galilean telescope in conjunction with an eye.*
   A. Object space
   B. Image space

d. Obviously, there are an infinite number of combinations of objective and ocular lens powers which will afford a given magnification. However, the length of the telescope will depend upon the relative focal lengths, higher power elements resulting in a shorter telescope. In an afocal telescope the length of the system is the algebraic sum of the focal lengths of the objective and the ocular.

B. Magnification produced by a telescopic system may also be evaluated by a comparison of the relative sizes of the entrance and exit pupils.

1. In most cases the entrance pupil of a Galilean telescope system is the objective. In those instances where this is not definite (where the objective lens is not the aperture stop) an artificial aperture stop can be added to the system by placing an opaque sheet of paper with a small aperture over the front of the objective lens. This aperture then becomes the entrance pupil.

2. The image of the objective formed by the ocular is the exit pupil of the telescope. When the objective is brightly illuminated this image appears as a luminous disc. It is called the *eye ring* or *Ramsden Circle*. In a Galilean telescope this image is located between the objective and ocular and thus is not available for exact measurement. However, it is possible to estimate its size accurately enough to result in relatively little error by holding a millimeter ruler in the apparent plane of the eye ring.

3. The formula for this expression of magnification is:

$$M = \frac{\text{Diameter of objective}}{\text{Diameter of eye ring}}$$

4. Southall (1933b) points out that this expression for angular magnification has the advantage that it is approximately true even if the telescope is not afocal. Error is introduced because the eye is not in the plane of the eye ring.

C. Still another method of determining the approximate magnification of focal telescopic systems may be employed when the internal specifications are known. The objective and ocular system are treated as thin lenses and the following formula utilized:

$$M = \left(\frac{1}{1-dF_1} \right) \left(\frac{1}{1-zF_v} \right)$$

where:

F_v = effective power of the telescope
F_1 = objective power
d = distance between average nodal points of objective and ocular
z = distance from ocular to eye

For afocal telescopes, $F_v = 0$, and the second component of the formula drops out leaving

$$M = \frac{1}{1-dF_1}$$

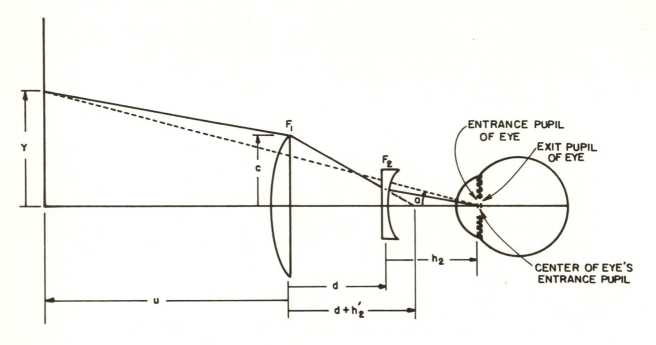

Fig. VI-22.   Field of view for a stationary eye with a Galilean telescope. (Westheimer, 1957).

D. Magnification of Telemicroscopes

Magnification produced by telescopic systems focused for near point distances may be analyzed in terms of angular (telescopic) magnification and relative distance magnification. The total magnification produced is the product of that produced individually by the two types of magnification.

e.g.:

A 2.0X telescope focused for 16.6 centimeters or 6.00 D. vergence may be evaluated in terms of 2.0X telescopic magnification and 6.00 D./4 = 1.5X relative distance magnification, relative to 25 centimeters. The total magnification denoted is (2.0X) (1.5X) equals 3.0X.

Field Of View

A. It is often stated that the field of view of a telescope is limited by its exit pupil.

   1. This assumes that the eye's entrance pupil is larger than the telescope's exit pupil and that their locations are coincident.

   2. Actually the eye's entrance pupil is usually smaller and the Galilean telescope's exit pupil is located within the instrument and thus coincidence of the pupils is not possible. In actual use, the eye's entrance pupil is usually the limiting factor.

   3. To maximize the field, the ocular should be as close to the eye as possible.

B. The size of the exit pupil of the telescope is dependent upon:

   1. The size of the objective

   2. The power of the ocular

   3. The distance between the objective and ocular

C. The diameter of the exit pupil may be determined by dividing the diameter of the objective lens by the magnifying power of the telescope.

D. The useable field size of a telescope may be reduced from the total field size due to aberration of lenses within the telescope.

E. In actual practice the field of view of a telescope may be specified in terms of degrees or in terms of the diameter of the circular view at a specific distance, usually 1000 yards. This latter specification is more likely to be found in the case of ready-made telescopes, monoculars, and binoculars.

F. Westheimer (1957) proposes the following formulae for the approximate field of view in object space of Galilean type telescopes using the eye's entrance pupil as the major reference point (based on thin lenses).

   1. For object at finite distance (see Figure VI-22)

$$Y = \frac{c(d + h'_2 - u)}{d + h'_2} + cF_1 u$$

where:

   Y = ½ linear extent of the object plane seen through the telescope
   c = ½ diameter of the objective lens (meters)
   d = distance between the objective and the ocular lenses (meters)
   h'_2 = distance from the ocular to the image of the eye's entrance pupil formed by the ocular
   F_1 = the power of the objective (including any near add)
   u = object distance from the objective lens

2. For object at infinity (see Figure VI-22)

$$\tan a = \frac{c}{M(h_2 M + D)}$$

   a = ½ angular extent of the field of view in object space
   c = ½ diameter of objective lens
   h_2 = distance from ocular lens to entrance pupil of the eye
   d = distance from objective to ocular
   M = magnification of the telescope

3. To determine the apparent field of view in image space (angle a') this formula must be multiplied by the magnification (M). Thus, for an object at infinity, the apparent field of view becomes:

$$\tan a' = M(\tan a) = \frac{c}{h_2 M + d}$$

G. As with microscopic lenses, the authors have found the easiest procedure for determining the practical field of view of a telescope is to view an object plane through the instrument and measure the extent of the field under the conditions of use.

Image Brightness

A. The image brightness of a telescope is determined by the size of the exit pupil relative to the size of the pupil of the eye.

B. In most cases, the exit pupil diameter is determined by the diameter of the objective lens system divided by the magnification power of the telescope.

   1. A 7 × 35 telescope designates 7× magnification and a 35 millimeter diameter objective and thus would have an exit pupil diameter of 5 mm. Hence a 5 mm. diameter bundle of light would reach the eye.

   2. There is no *brightness* advantage in having a telescopic exit pupil larger than the pupil of the eye. The images seen through 7 × 35 mm. and 7 × 50 mm. telescopes will appear equally bright *if* the eye's pupil is 5 mm. diameter or less in both cases.

C. Relative Light Efficiency is calculated by squaring the exit pupil diameter. When coated optics are used, 50 percent is added.

D. Since low vision patients generally are especially sensitive to illumination, this quality of telescopes is important in selecting the proper telescope for a particular patient, especially when more than one type is available in the same magnification range.

E. Having determined the required magnification, to select the optimum telescope for brightness for a particular patient, one must consider the patient's light requirement, the conditions of use (photopic or scotopic) and the eye's pupil size under these conditions.

   1. A glaucoma patient with a constant 2 mm. pupil size and requiring maximum light will receive no increase in brightness from a 6 × 50 compared to a 6 × 15 whether day or night.

   2. A patient who is in need of a bright image who has a 2mm. pupil in daylight but a 5 mm. pupil at night would find the 6 × 15 telescope satisfactory in daylight, but a 6 × 30 better at night. However, a 6 × 50 would not further improve the image brightness for him.

Accommodation and Telescopes

A. Because of the optics of a telescopic system, the demand on accommodation to view a near object through the telescope is much greater than would be indicated by the object distance (see Figure VI-23).

B. Freid (1973) has derived the following formula for estimation of accommodation required at the ocular lens when a near object is viewed through an afocal telescope composed of thin lenses:

$$A_{oc} = \frac{M^2 U}{1-dMU}$$

where:

   A_{oc} = accommodation at ocular
   M = magnification of telescope
   U = object vergence at objective
   d = distance (meters) from objective to ocular (positive)

For spectacle telescopes, where d is usually quite small, a very close approximation of the accommodative stimulus through the telescope can be made by multiplying the object vergence by

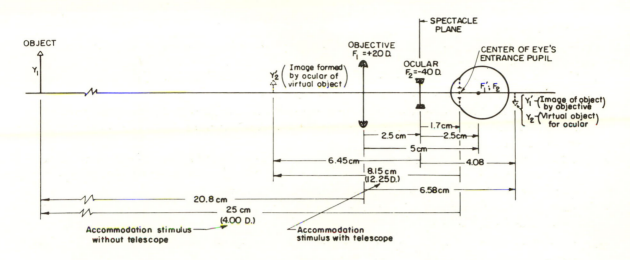

Fig. VI-23. *Diagram showing locations of images formed by an afocal Galilean telescope for a near object.*

The real object (Y₁) is located 25cm. in front of the eye. The objective (F₁) converges the rays from this object as if to form a real image (Y₁') 6.58cm. behind the objective. This image (Y₁') becomes a virtual object (Y₂) for the ocular (F₂) which is 2.5cm. behind the objective. Thus, Y₁' and Y₂ are 4.08cm. behind the ocular (F₂). The ocular diverges the rays to produce a virtual image (Y₂') 6.45cm. in front of the ocular. This image becomes the object viewed by the eye and is located 8.15cm. in front of the eye, thus requiring 12.25D. of accommodation. Note that the original real object (Y₁) when viewed without the telescope only requires 4.00D. of accommodation.

the square of the magnification ($A_{oc} = M^2U$).

C. It is apparent from Figure VI-24 that objects closer than one meter from the telescope specified will put a greater demand on accommodation than that which the average pre-presbyope can sustain. For object distance of ¾ meter or less, adequate accommodation cannot be maintained except by the very young. For the designs commonly used, as the magnification of telescopes increases, the effectivity of accommodation through them decreases markedly. From the above formula, it is apparent that the demand on accommodation is approximately directly proportional to the *square* of the magnification. Hence, a 4× or stronger telescope focused for infinity will require an insupportable amount of accommodation to focus even at 10 feet except for the very young.

D. In view of the above, to use a telescope for near object distances, it is necessary to eliminate some if not all of the requirements on accommodation.

1. This can be accomplished by changing the distance between the objective and ocular systems or by adding convex lens power to either system. For near viewing distances, the method of choice is addition of convex lens powers. For intermediate and far viewing distances, increasing the objective to ocular distance is the method of choice. While sportoculars use the latter method, prescription spectacle telescopes are made with unvarying length and thus rely on the former method.

2. Because the added power needed at the objective system is less than that required at the ocular system for the same effect, the convex power is usually added to the former, sometimes in the form of a "reading cap" which slides over the objective end of the telescope.

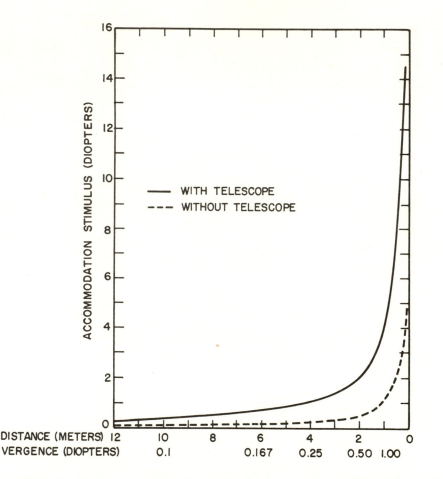

Fig. VI-24.   *Graph of accommodative stimulus as a function of object distance with and without a telescope. The calculations assumed a 2X afocal Galilean telescope with an objective to ocular distance of 2.5cm., with all measurements referred to the plane of the ocular.*

   Note that for the customary 3 meter low vision examination test distance, the accommodative stimulus is increased from a neglible 0.33D. to 1.30D. This difference increases greatly at the shorter object distances. Had the graph been plotted for a telescope of a greater magnification the discrepancies in accommodative stimuli would have been even more striking.

3. The "reading add" used is usually equal to the vergence distance of the object from the objective lens. Hence, the object is in the primary focal plane of the "reading add" lens and light leaves this lens (and enters the telescope objective) as parallel rays.

Ametropia Correction And Telescopes
A. The correction of refractive errors while using a telescope *may* be accomplished by varying the distance between the objective and ocular as discussed previously.

B. Because of its simplicity and directness ametropia corrections are usually added behind the ocular system of a fixed focus telescope. Only in this location is the power of the added lens equal in amount to the actual ametropia.

Aberrations in Telescopes

A. Because of their restricted field of view, peripheral aberrations inherent in the objectives of telescopes are not as important as in the oculars or in microscopic lenses.

B. Objectives of telescopes are usually designed with emphasis on the reduction of spherical aberration, coma, and axial chromatic aberrations (Sears, 1948).

C. Oculars of telescopes require correction for the same aberrations as microscopic lenses with particular emphasis on lateral chromatic aberration (Jenkins and White, 1957).

Chapter 7

The Low Vision Examination

Introduction

Many of the techniques used in the low vision examination are the same as those used in other optometric routines. These will not be given great emphasis here. However, many techniques do differ and these will be emphasized. The examination is ideally performed in at least two visits. This permits seeing the patient under different circumstances and giving the patient time to consider some of the findings and some of his desires between visits. A tentative prescription decided upon at the end of the first visit is seldom that which is finally ordered.

General Observations

Much can be learned by careful observation of the patient.

Mobility

A. Does he walk with help or by himself? It is often a good practice to place some obstacle in the patient's path and observe how he gets around it.

B. Does he use a cane? Is it used as a sign to others of his handicap; as a physical support; or as a substitute for vision?

C. Does the patient appear to grope for things or easily recognize doorways and similar obstacles?

Posture

A. How does he hold his head? Is it held down to avoid a bright light?
B. Does he look where he is going? Does he look at people with whom he converses?

Fixation

A. Does the patient have centric or marked eccentric fixation?

B. Is there a nystagmus?

Cosmesis

What is the cosmetic appearance of the patient's eyes: ptosis, scars, etc.?

Physical Factors

A. Does the patient have any other obvious handicaps such as hearing loss, paralysis or problems in locomotion?

B. Does he exhibit a tremor?

C. Does the patient appear feeble or in robust health?

Psychological Factors

A. Does the patient appear independent or does he rely on some other member of the family for mobility and decisions?

B. Does the patient exhibit efficient mental function?

C. What is general attitude: resigned, rebellious, aggressive, depressed, inadequate, expectant, eager, ambitious, etc.?

Case History

Duration

How long has the condition of low vision been present? A longer duration indicates a better prognosis for a successful patient.

Stability

Has there been any recent change in vision? When? A stable condition is desirable. If the condition is active, a medical consultation is indicated and consideration should be given to the prognosis.

Etiology

A. *What does the patient think is the cause of the vision loss?*

B. *What other doctors has he seen? What have they told him?* Do not elicit too much detail. This can be both time consuming and depressing for the patient. The patient may need sympathy and encouragement at this point, but the practitioner must always be careful not to over-promise.

Education

A. *What was the extent of the education?*

B. *Was the patient educated in regular schools and classes, in a blind institution, or with special assistance?*

C. *Did he use large print, or Braille?*

Occupation

A. *Previous to vision loss?*
B. *Present occupation?*
C. *Aspirations?*
D. *Avocations?*

Mobility

Can the patient get around <u>alone</u> in strange places?
A. *Indoors? Outdoors?*

B. *By sight or by touch?*

This is indicative of the extent of the visual field. A patient who has a nearly normal peripheral field and a macula lesion should be able to get around outdoors alone in strange places. A patient who can get around indoors but not outdoors probably exhibits a form field constriction.

Visual Performance

A. *Is vision better in daylight or twilight? Does the patient wear sunglasses or shade his eyes outdoors?*

If vision is worse in bright light, it is indicative of either a media involvement or cone damage with mostly rod vision remaining. Lowered vision in dim light may be indicative of impaired rod function.

B. *Does he see street signs or house numbers? Can he recognize the number on a bus? Can he cross streets alone, watching signals or other people?*

C. *Does he attend movies? Watch TV? What viewing distance?*

Present Aids

A. *When was the last refraction? What was prescribed? For what purpose?*

B. *What prescription or prescriptions are presently being used?*

C. *What magnifying aids are owned? Which are presently being used? For what purpose?*

Motivation

For what purpose does the patient express a desire to see better? Is motivation mild, moderate or strong? Specific tasks should be elicited rather than generalizations like wanting "to see better".

Examination Procedures

Ophthalmoscopy, External Examination, Biomicroscopy, and Pupillary Reflexes

These tests are performed in the usual manner although they may present difficulties. In performing them, the practitioner is looking for the cause of the low vision, verifying the history that the patient has given, and attempting to determine whether the condition is arrested or active. If the condition is active, consideration should immediately be given to referral for medical diagnosis and treatment unless one is aware that the patient is currently under active care. In this case, wherever practical, attempts should be made to consult the other doctor involved for an exchange of information. It is important to determine if the pathology is of a type that is apt to be progressive and if so how rapidly.

The major consideration in terms of assisting low vision patients is the determination of the areas that are affected and unaffected. Which areas of the retina appear the most useable? Are there opacities of the media? Is the cornea badly damaged? These considerations will point the direction that low vision aids may take.

The most important thing is not to be discouraged by appearances or reports. For example, it is easy to jump to the unwarranted conclusion that the entire macula area has been destroyed, when actually some cones may have survived and can be used with high illumination. Many eyes that have media so opacified that the examiner cannot *see in*, are not so opacified that the patient cannot *"see out"*.

Retinoscopy

If possible, standard retinoscopy should be done *using a trial frame* so that the patient may turn his head in any direction and so that we may examine along any axis on which a reflex is visible. If standard retinoscopy is impossible, radical retinoscopy, where the working distance is decreased until a recognizable reflex is seen, should be used. In media involvements where the usual technique does not produce a useful reflex, off axis retinoscopy may be possible.

Because of uncertainties of fixation, media involvements, and irregularities of the refracting surfaces, retinoscopy may be somewhat unreliable. One cannot assume the reversibility of a selected light path. The axis along which retinoscopy is performed may not be the axis which the patient favors for fixation or which produces his best acuity.

Keratometry

This is performed in the usual manner and may be helpful in cases of high astigmia or in revealing an irregularity of the corneal surface.

Visual Field Studies

It is often helpful to have information concerning the extent of the visual field and the size and extent of any scotomas present. One must, of course, use large enough targets and a large enough fixation object for the patient to see. For some patients, the Amsler Grid may produce more critical information on the integrity of the macular and para-macular areas.

In many instances there exists a central scotoma which causes an additional problem in fixation. If a large cross is drawn upon the tangent screen centering on the fixation target and a large circle is drawn upon the screen with the fixation point at its center, the patient can then be instructed to watch the point at the center of the circle where the cross lines would intersect (see Figure VII-1). This will, in most instances, provide adequate fixation even with a central scotoma.

Many apparently paradoxical visual difficulties are explicable and soluble when the nature of the visual fields is known. For example, a scotoma, extending to the right of the preferred fixation area, may cause reading difficulties inconsistent with the patient's ability to discriminate small type (see Figure IV-5). Or the eye with much poorer corrected acuity may be the one which is capable of the better overall performance.

Color Vision Testing

Color vision is a product of cone vision and thus becomes a sensitive method of determining the extent of damage to the central retinal area and the optic nerve serving it, even on occasions when the fundi cannot be visualized.

Standard pseudo-isochromatic plate tests are not suitable for testing acquired color vision defects or for testing partially-sighted subjects requiring high contrast. The Farnsworth Panel D-15 test (see Figure IV-4) can be quickly administered and easily scored even with partially-sighted subjects (Adams, et al., 1974).

When checking for acquired color vision defects, the test should be performed on each eye separately. A Macbeth lamp or a *daylight* fluorescent lamp should be used as the illuminant.

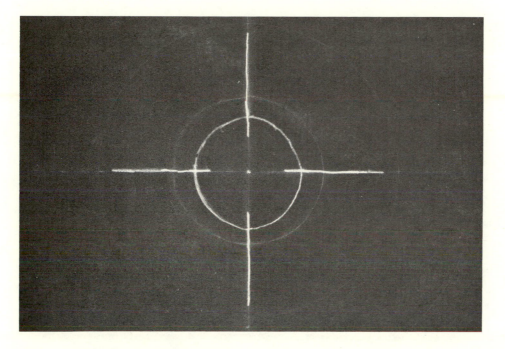

Fig. VII-1. Tangent screen fixation target for use with a large central scotoma.

Subjective Testing, Success Oriented Procedures

This is the heart of the low vision examination. It is here that the psychological factors in the examination can become most important. Every attempt should be made to *encourage* rather than *discourage* the patient. This should be a *success oriented examination*.

The tempo of the examination should be kept slow enough for the patient to follow instructions, without a feeling of frustration.

A. Equipment

1. Distance charts should be available with letters up to 700 or 800 foot Snellen notation. The Designs for Vision distance test chart by William Feinbloom has numbers up to 700 feet (see Figure VII-2). The gradations should be fine enough to measure acuities in the ranges *between* 400 and 300, 300 and 200, and 200 and 100. Below 200 feet the Bausch and Lomb No. 713591, AMA Ratings chart (see Figure VII-3) and the Louise Sloan Charts made by Good Lite Company (see Figure VII-4) meet these requirements.

For children or illiterates, hand held E cards or the New York Lighthouse picture symbol flash cards are useful (see Figure VII-5).

Means should be available to hold large charts at ten feet or closer and to vary the illumination upon them.

2. Near point charts *should be available in great variety*. They should afford a very large range of type sizes and spacings between characters. There should be isolated characters and groups of characters as well as paragraphs. All printing should be clear and of good contrast.

Message charts should be carefully screened. All messages should be neutral or psychologically

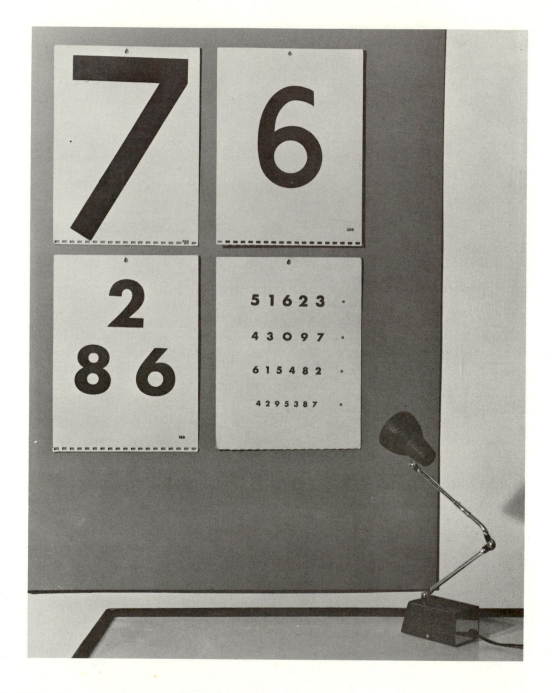

Fig. VII-2. *Distance test chart arranged by William Feinbloom, D. D. The four pages shown include foot letter sizes: 700; 350; 180; and 40, 30, 25, and 20. The complete chart also includes pages of digits of foot letter sizes: 600; 400; 300; 205; 200; 160; 140; 120; and 100, 80, and 60. (Reproduced by permission of Designs for Vision, Inc.)*

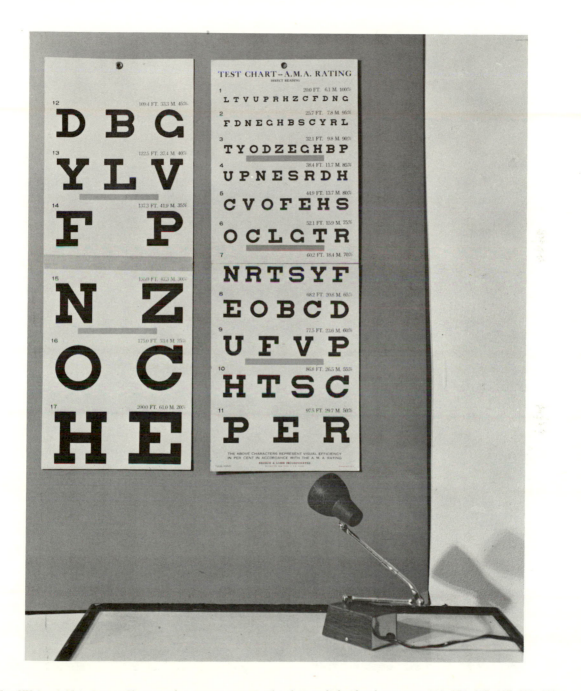

Fig. VII-3.   A.M.A. Rating Chart number 713591-101ND. The chart includes foot letter sizes: 200, 175, 155, 137, 122, 109, 97, 87, 77, 68, 60, 52, 45, 38, 32, 26, and 20. The chart also has red, green, and blue lines which can be used for a gross color recognition test. (Reproduced by permission of Bausch and Lomb, Inc.)

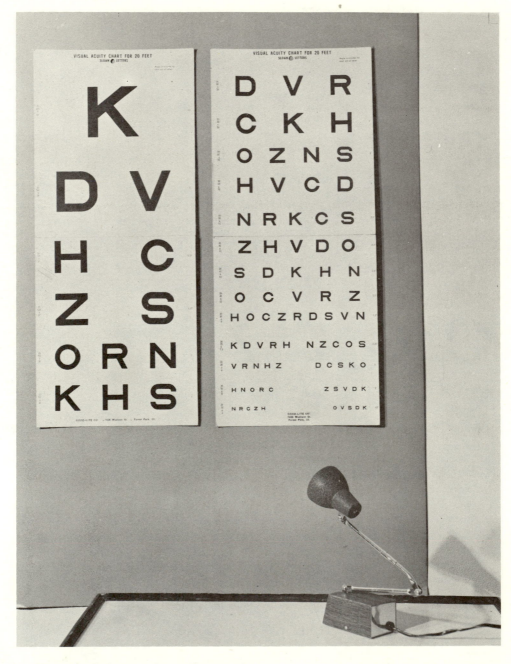

Fig. VII-4.   Louise Sloan's distance test chart. The chart includes foot letter sizes: 200, 160, 125, 100, 80, 60, 50, 40, 30, 25, 20, 16, and 13. (Reproduced by permission of Good-lite Co.)

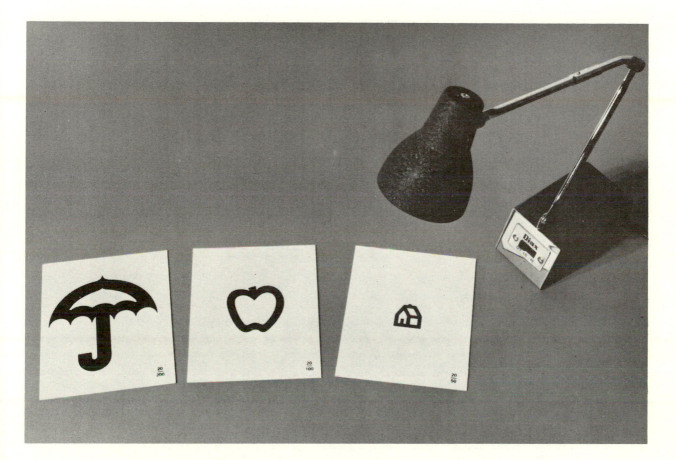

Fig. VII-5.   The New York Lighthouse picture symbol flash cards after Schering. The three symbols are repeated for each of the following foot letter sizes: 200, 100, 50, 40, 30, 20, 15, 10. (Reproduced by permission of The New York Association for the Blind.)

appropriate for the partially-sighted. For example, cards containing thoughts such as "next to life itself, God's most precious gift is sight" should never be used in a low vision examination.

a. The Feinbloom chart of numbers by Designs for Vision (see Figure VII-6A) is unique and practically indispensable. It has a range from 4 point to 24 point type, consisting of carefully spaced isolated and grouped numerals.

b. The Hoff chart and the Feinbloom message chart (see Figure VII-6B) contain messages appropriate for encouraging and instructing the partially-sighted.

c. The Lebensohn chart (Lebensohn, 1936) has a range from 2 point to 24 point type with many gradations and varied characters.

d. *Stimson's Optical Aids for Low Acuity* (1957) contains a number of good near point charts.

e. The N. H. Howard card (1959) contains examples of printed matter encountered in everyday living, i.e., typewriting, stock quotations, telephone directory, newsprint, etc.

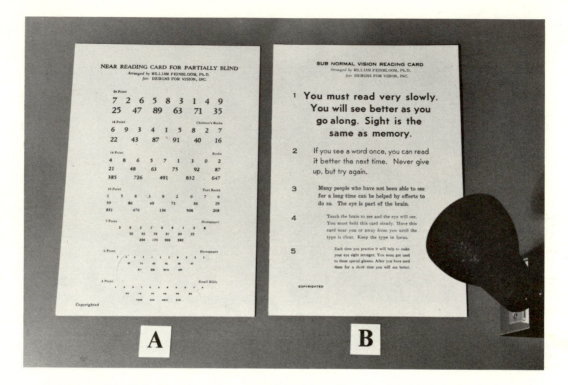

Fig. VII-6. Near reading cards by William Feinbloom, O.D. (Reproduced by permission of Designs For Vision, Inc.).

A. Number card arranged with single, double, triple, and quadruple digits. This card is especially useful for determining the effect of contour interaction.

B. Message chart with text for the partially-sighted. The type sizes are: 2.75M, 2.0M, 1.4M, 1.25M, and 1.0M. This card may be more easily read than others having the same size type because of the spacing.

f. The Sloan Reading Cards (Sloan and Brown, 1963) are textual matter graded according to M ratings from 1 M to 10 M (see Figure VII-7).

g. The American Optical Company chart #11970 contains textual material from 2 M to 0.5 M.

h. The American Optical Company chart #11960 consists of 13 lines of illiterate E's graded from 14/14 to 14/224.

i. The New York Lighthouse has a near vision test card for children using the same three picture symbols as their hand held distance flash cards. The sizes range from 8 M through 0.5 M (see Figure VII-8).

j. Many other good cards are available, which meet the discussed criteria, besides those listed above.

3. Trial frame and trial lens sets are the preferred equipment for the low vision examination. This makes it possible for the patient to fixate eccentrically and for the examiner to *observe* the

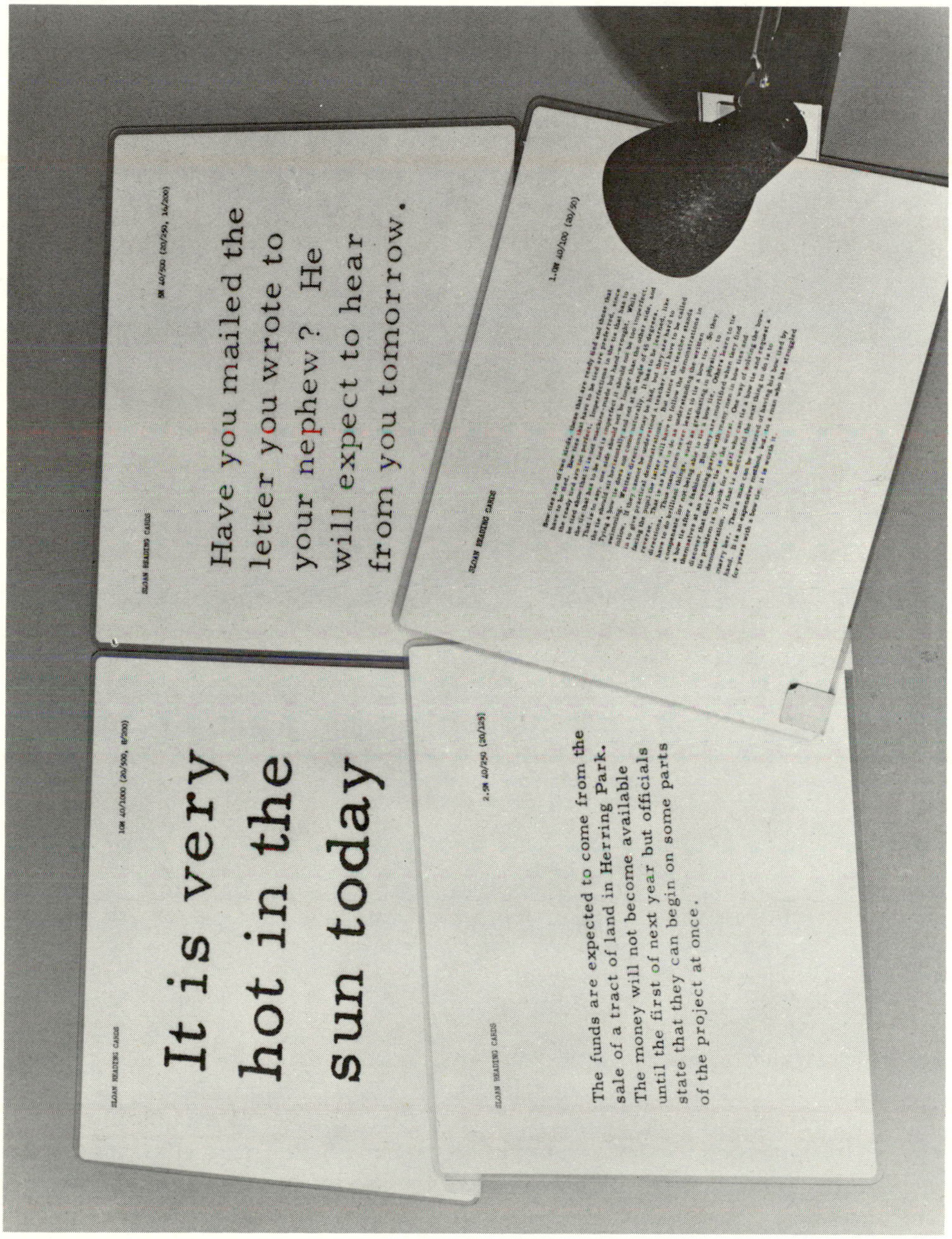

Fig. VII-7.   *Sloan Reading Cards. The series is composed of type sizes: 10M, 7M, 5M, 4M, 3M, 2.5M, 2.0M, 1.5M, and 1M. The larger sizes are especially useful for evaluating reading ability at cutomary reading distances using relative size magnification without introducing the complications of strong magnifiers and precise shortened working distances. (Reproduced by permission of Louise Sloan, Ph.D.).*

NEAR VISION TEST
SYMBOLS FOR CHILDREN

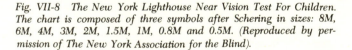

			DISTANT EQUIVALENT	METER SIZE
			20/400	8M
			20/300	6M
			20/200	4M
			20/160	3M 27 Pt.
			20/100	2M 18 Pt.
			20/80	1.5M 14 Pt.
			20/50	1M 9 Pt.
			20/40	.8M 7 Pt.
			20/25	.5M 4 Pt.

18 Point Large Type Grades 1-3
14 Point Average Book Print Grades 4-7
9 Point Magazines, Paper Back Books, Typing
7 Point Newspaper

Distance equivalent calibrated for 40 cm (16 inches)

THE LIGHTHOUSE LOW VISION SERVICES
111 EAST 59th STREET, NEW YORK, N.Y. 10022   ©1970   LLV-2

Fig. VII-8   The New York Lighthouse Near Vision Test For Children. The chart is composed of three symbols after Schering in sizes: 8M, 6M, 4M, 3M, 2M, 1.5M, 1M, 0.8M and 0.5M. (Reproduced by permission of The New York Association for the Blind).

manner in which the patient is fixating, the alterations in nystagmus, squinting, head tilt, etc. Rapid comparisons of widely separated lens powers, in the steps desired, are more readily performed with the trial frame than with the phoroptor. The simple equipment also, as William Feinbloom (1960) has pointed out, creates in the patient a better sense of reality and leaves him with a greater confidence in the performance of *his own eyes* as opposed to some wondrous and imposing machine.

The trial frame should be adjustable and sturdy and permit a near-point chart to be held at a very close distance. A corrected curve lens set allows the insertion of more high power lenses into adjacent cells of the trial frame. It also results in fewer aberrations, however in some powers the smaller lens aperture may cause difficulties.

4. Hand flip cross-cylinders of ± 0.50 D. and ± 1.00 D. are useful.

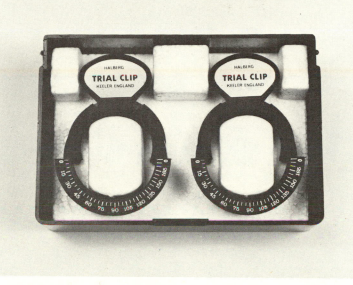

Fig. VII-9.   Halberg Trial Clips. These spring loaded clips, each having two lens cells, are especially useful for over-refraction.

5. Halberg trial clips made by Keeler Optical are extremely helpful for improvising a child's trial frame and for adding lenses over existing spectacles (see Figure VII-9).

6. T. R. Kuhns has designed a "near vision screener" which is essentially a 15 centimeter pocket ruler marked one side in inches, centimeters, and diopters. The other side contains print rated from 6 M through 0.35 M and a small equivalent type size table (see Figure VII-10). It is available from the New York Lighthouse.

7. An assortment of illumination controls should be available. A floor stand goose-neck lamp is most beneficial for variable lighting on all charts. Typoscopes, visors, side shields, tinted lenses etc. should also be available.

8. Some type of stand for supporting near reading material may be required. A table easel serves this purpose (see Figure VII-11).

9. Various powers of microscopic and telescopic trial lenses, hand and stand magnifiers, and hand held telescopes are needed.

B. Procedures

The starting point should be the prescription that the examiner feels has the best chance of providing good acuity, whether this is the retinoscopy or the previous prescription. It is best to start binocularly or with the better eye. Even though the patient may claim that the poorer eye is useless, some attempt should be made to test it later.

For psychological impact, the *first* attempt to read a chart should meet with *success*. It is therefore advisable to start with the largest available letter at a distance of ten feet, unless there is reason to believe a closer distance is necessary. In this way the patient will not be immediately presented with another failure.

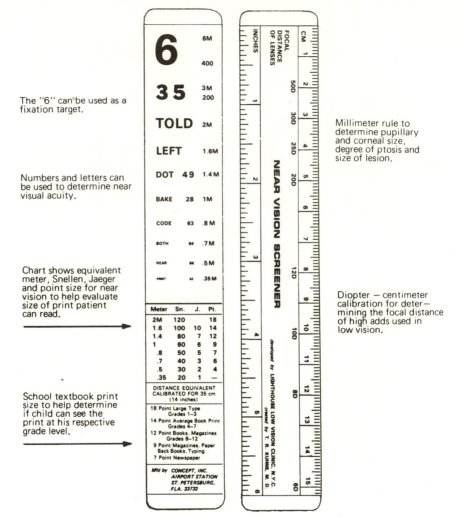

NEAR VISION SCREENER

The "6" can be used as a fixation target.

Numbers and letters can be used to determine near visual acuity.

Chart shows equivalent meter, Snellen, Jaeger and point size for near vision to help evaluate size of print patient can read.

School textbook print size to help determine if child can see the print at his respective grade level.

Millimeter rule to determine pupillary and corneal size, degree of ptosis and size of lesion.

Diopter — centimeter calibration for deter—mining the focal distance of high adds used in low vision.

Fig. VII-10. Kuhns' Near Vision Screener. (Reproduced by permission of Concept, Inc.)

Although any distance may be used for testing, the 10 foot distance has advantages. The rating obtained is, of course, *recorded* in terms of the *distance of the test* as well as the *size of the letter*, e.g. 10/120. (By multiplying by 2 it can easily be converted to its more familiar 20 ft. equivalent.) The shorter distance has the advantage of making all the testing charts appear twice as large and many patients who have been discouraged because they could not read the charts in the doctor's office (where the largest test unit was probably 20/200 or at best 20/400) now find that they are able to read several lines of the low vision chart.

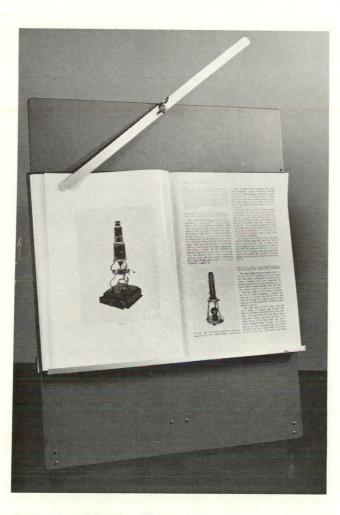

Fig. VII-11.   Adjustable reading stand and table easel manufactured
by Testrite Instrument Co., Inc.

Better acuity ratings are obtained by progressing from the readable to the unreadable rather than conversely. The improved performance encourages the patients to continue and try for further achievement. The encouraging attitude of the examiner should also reinforce this atmosphere of success.

The dioptric steps in testing must be large enough to elicit recognition of a difference. One diopter steps are frequently used but even larger intervals may be tried. It is possible to refine a prescription to a half diopter, by bracketing, even though two diopter intervals are being used in the subjective comparisons.

Where very low acuity is elicited, large jumps and large extremes of prescription should be tried. Plus and minus 5, 10, or even 20 diopter lenses, may elicit a favorable response and produce a start on a subjective examination in an unsuspected refractive region.

Unless they appear to improve acuity, cylindrical corrections may be ignored. Often, large cylindrical corrections may be found, which do not improve acuity at all. An astigmatic correction which makes a significant difference should be recorded. It is well to remember that the discrimination of the patient may be lowered by his visual defect and subjective testing may give a wide variety of responses. When this appears to be the case it is wise to check the final astigmatic correction obtained against the purely spherical correction or a smaller correction previously worn.

The test for astigmatism is most easily performed with the flip cross-cylinder in the usual manner. It is only necessary to remember that a sufficiently large cross-cylinder must be used so the patient can differentiate between the two positions offered. The letters fixated must also be sufficiently large to be distinguished even with the addition of a cross-cylinder of one diopter. In some instances, the best method of determining the axis of the cylinder is by rotating the cylindrical lens until a blur is reported. The rotation is then reversed until a blur is again noted. The cylinder axis should then be the mid-point between the two reported blurs.

For irregular astigmatism, the stenopaic slit may be used with spheres to test the principle meridians. Borish (1970) outlines the procedure very clearly.

Illumination Evaluations

With the best distance correction in the trial frame variation of illumination should be tried. Increasing or decreasing the illumination on the chart may have a dramatic effect. The incidence of extraneous light upon the eyes of the patient, particularly in cases of opacities of the media, may also have a marked effect. The result of inserting a visor to shade the eyes of the patient from overhead illumination should be noted. Side shields may also be tried and their effect noted.

Telescopic Testing

A. Whenever a telescopic spectacle is considered or when it is desired to further refine the subjective correction, testing can be performed through a telescopic system. 1.7× TS or 2.2× TS are the usual lens systems for this purpose, the 2.2× being the most commonly used. Since the telescope is an afocal instrument, the *best* distance correction (sphere and cylinder) must be incorporated into the trial frame before the telescope is inserted. This prescription is put into the rear rings and the telescope in the next free ring anterior to the refractive correction.

The telescope testing requires that the other eye be occluded. In most instances a frosted glass is preferable to a black disc.

In aligning the telescope, the height, lateral displacement, and tilt must all be taken into consideration. Ideally, the optical axis of the telescope should be coincident with the extension of the visual axis of the eye as it fixates the chart. Often, the best way of aligning the telescope is subjectively.

The patient may require some orientation in finding the chart with the reduced visual field and greater magnification. It is expected that a 2× telescope will double the apparent size of the letters and hence the patient should now be able to read a letter half the size of the smallest letter previously resolved. This theoretical consideration is not always borne out. Sometimes a smaller increase is obtained and, surprisingly, sometimes a much greater increase is obtained. Partly, this greater increase in performance may be attributed to the fact that not only are the letters enlarged but also the spaces around them. It is typical of patients using non-foveal fixation that their acuity is enhanced by wider separation of the characters being discriminated. The same characteristic of eccentrically fixating amblyopes has been noted by Flom (1966) and attributed to contour interaction.

In modifying the subjective correction with the telescope in place, any correction lens must be placed behind the telescope rather than in front of it. This applies to both spherical and cylindrical lenses as well as the flip cross-cylinder, and while it does create slight mechanical difficulties, it can be done. It is important that the telescope be accurately aligned, otherwise an astigmatic error can be introduced from the tilting of the telescope.

Frequently, the modified correction of the refractive error, determined with the telescope in place, will be found to be better, even when the telescope has been removed, than the subjective determination made without the use of the telescope. However, in most cases the telescopic correction will result in more convex lens power than the non-telescopic correction because of the great increase in vergence of rays (from an object at a finite distance) when passing through a telescope (see Chapter VI, OPTICS: Telescopes, *Accommodation and Telescopes*). In routine examinations one generally ignores the 0.33 D. vergence involved in a 10 ft. test distance. However, a $2\times$ telescope with a lens aperture of 2.0 cm. changes the 0.33 D. vergence at the objective to 1.34 D. vergence at the ocular.

B. If it is desired, a telescope of different power may be tried, particularly if a prescription of this type is deemed possible. Because of aberrations and other factors it is not always possible to predict the performance obtainable with a different power telescope from that obtained with one of greater or lesser magnification.

C. Where there is sufficient useable vision in the other eye, it should also be tested with a telescope.

Binocular testing is possible, but very difficult and time consuming. The two telescopes must be of the same power and the tubes must be in perfect alignment with each other and both aligned so that their axes meet at the chart.

D. Because of the high demands placed on accommodation even for fixation distances of ten or twenty feet, and because of increased aberrations resulting in very small fields of view, the practical limit of fixed focus telescopic spectacles for distance viewing is usually considered to be $3\times$. When greater magnification than this is required, testing can be continued with hand held focusable telescopes of $4\times$, $6\times$, $8\times$, and $10\times$.

Many patients will require assistance in focusing and aiming strong telescopes. The usual focusing mechanism involves the ocular, however, with many of these telescopes the focusing range can be increased by unscrewing the objective.

Near Testing

A. The Systematic Approach

Near point testing is extremely important since the greatest benefit of low vision care is often the enhancement of close vision. The primary consideration is *how much* a patient can see, *not* what he can see at a *fixed distance*.

There are many methods of conducting the near point examination. The important thing is to have a *systematic*, rather than a hit and miss approach.

B. Calculations of an add based on the distance acuity

1. Assuming that the formula for effective magnification (M = F/4) is to be used, then the

magnification obtained from a convex lens equals the dioptric power divided by 4. If one assumes that the patient will be well served if he has the equivalent of 20/40 acuity for near (this would enable him to read the usual type of newsprint with some reserve) then one can calculate the magnification required to enlarge the retinal image of a 40 foot letter to the same size as the retinal image of the letter that can be seen by this patient at twenty feet.

2. e.g.

Distance acuity = 20/200
Near requirement = 20/40
Required M = 200/40 = 5×
M = F/4
5 = F/4
F = +20.00
Print must be 5 cm. from the lenses.

This lens power becomes a starting point for the subjective examination at near.

3. These calculations assume a number of things.

a. One of these, is that the patient is not exercising any of his own accommodation. Any accommodation used by the patient should be subtracted to modify the correction for near.

b. The calculated lens power is, of course, to be added to the previously obtained distance refractive correction. These should be combined into the least number of lenses possible. For strong adds and low acuities, cylindrical corrections up to approximately two diopters can usually be omitted initially. Hence, if the distance correction is +3.00 D. and the calculated magnification required for close work is 5× (+20.00 D.), the first lens tried should be approximately +23.00 D. in power. Practically, this might mean a 6× lens (+24.00 D.)

C. Calculations of an add based on a near point test

1. Many examiners prefer to test the acuity on graded test types at some fixed distance. Forty centimeters is usually considered "sacred" unto the gods of optics! If the "equivalent" acuity at forty centimeters is 20/200 (0.40/4.0 M) and it is desired that the patient be able to read the "equivalent" 20/40 (0.8 M) type, the print must be held at one-fifth the distance or at eight centimeters. It is now possible to calculate the lens or accommodative power required to focus at eight centimeters, this being +12.50 D. Again this must be added to the distance correction.

2. In the initial testing at forty centimeters it may be necessary to use up to a +2.50 D. add, if the patient is presbyopic.

3. The calculated add (+12.50 D.) plus the distance correction (+3.00 D. in the example) or a total of +15.50 D. becomes the starting point for the near examination.

D. Comparison of the two methods.

It is obvious that the calculations using distance acuity and the formula M = F/4 result in a greater lens power to achieve the magnification than the method of calculating the required reading distance based on measuring the acuity at forty centimeters. Often the final prescription will fall somewhere between these two calculations.

Those advocating the second method believe that the patient should be led from larger type at greater distance towards smaller type at a lesser distance. On the other hand, those advocating trying the greater lens power first feel there is a great psychological gain when the patient is immediately shown a lens which permits him to read very small type. Certainly, with the patient who requires encouragement, it is better to begin with too much lens power rather than risk his frustration by using too little.

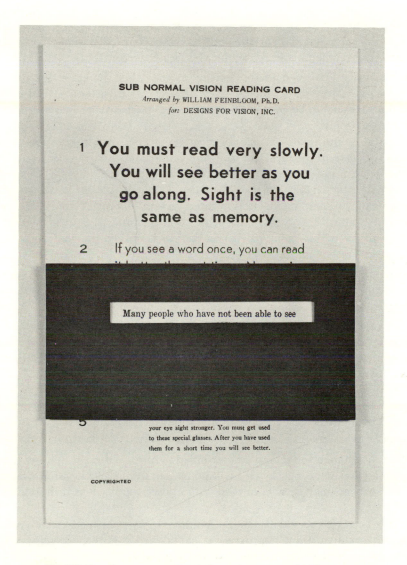

Fig. VII-12.   *Typoscope used to isolate print to be read. (Chart reproduced by permission of Designs For Vision, Inc.)*

E. Refinement of the near point lens prescription.

1. With high power lenses, it is extremely important that the patient look through the optical center, and that the visual axis be perpendicular to the lens surfaces and the reading card. This requires that the trial frame be carefully adjusted to the patient's face with regard to vertical and lateral centration as well as tilt and vertex distance. In addition, the reading card is positioned directly in front of the eye and lens (instead of the usual inferior position) and held parallel to the lens plane.

2. In near point testing with strong convex lenses it is important to keep illumination on the test card and to be sure that the patient realizes which line he is expected to read. For this purpose a typoscope (reading mask) is very helpful (see Figure VII-12).

3. Patients will usually tend to hold the reading card at their habitual distance and must be encouraged to bring it closer, even though they protest that they do not read at *that* distance. The expected distance should be calculated and the card placed there initially. The patient may then adjust it for best focus.

When the card is at its optimum distance for clear vision the patient is started on reading large print, to encourage his performance and to assure immediate success. The Feinbloom (Designs for Vision) number card is excellent for this purpose (see Figure VII-6A). The single widely spaced numbers are much easier to read than the double, triple, or quadruple numbers and these in turn are easier to read than closely printed type in sentence form.

When the patient is able to read the large print he is encouraged to read smaller and smaller type. If he can perform with 4 point type (!) on this card, he then proceeds to a card containing sentences, and again starts with the large size type.

4. When the finest print that the patient can read with the initial lens has been determined one is ready to try other powers. If the patient has been able to read extremely fine type such as 5 or 6 point sentences, then one should try lenses of lower power. If the patient has not been able to read the finest type on the card one should try lenses of higher power.

Even though the patient may be able to read the very finest print with greater facility, it is better to determine the *lowest* power lens that permits reading of the *smallest* print. If some special requirements are known, such as the reading of music, this may be tried although generally it would be reserved for the second examination.

5. Before a final lens power is recorded, a determination should be made of the effect of any previously found cylindrical correction. While low power cylinders may frequently be omitted, often strong power cylinders may be reduced when combined with a strong spherical element.

6. As in the case of distance refraction, a determination of the effect of lighting should be made by trying low, high and very high levels of illumination. Often a low vision patient, if there is partial cone impairment, may be able to read with a lower power lens if illumination levels are very high.

The effect of the typoscope should also be determined. In cases of media involvement, it can be very dramatic when a significant improvement is obtained simply by placing a typoscope on the reading material to reduce reflections from the surrounding paper.

7. The near visual acuity and also the reading ability of the patient with various lenses should be recorded. Different systems of type notation were discussed in Chapter 5.

If points or Jaeger are used, they should be recorded with the working distance and the chart or type of material read.

e.g., Feinbloom 4 point single digits @ 10 cm.

This indicates that double or multiple digits, and certainly sentences of that size could *not* be read. (The ability or inability to read sentences printed in larger type should also be noted.) If M notation is used, a Snellen fraction can be written in meters.

e.g., 0.15/0.50 M sentences with good facility.

In all cases notation should be made of the illumination level and controls.

F. Near point testing with a telescopic spectacle

1. If the magnification using a telescope appears to be within a practical range, near point tests with the telescope should be considered. Magnification through the telescope for near is determined by multiplying the magnification of the distance telescope by the magnification of the reading cap added on the *front* of the telescope.

e.g.

$$M \text{ (distance)} = 2.2\times$$
$$\text{Near add} = +8.00 \text{ D.}$$
$$M \text{ (add)} = F/4 = +8.00/4 = 2\times$$
$$M \text{ (total)} = (2.2)(2) = 4.4\times$$

2. The practical limit of adds on telescopic spectacles is approximately $+10.00$ D. This means that the limit of magnification with a $2.2\times$ TS and a $+10.00$ D. add is $5.5\times$. A $6\times$ magnification could be obtained using a $3.0\times$ TS with a $+8.00$ D. add.

3. In using a telescopic, the magnification required for near can be calculated from the visual acuity at distance without the telescopic and the necessary equivalent acuity at near (as explained in Near Testing above). This total telescopic magnification determines the possible combinations of distance telescopes and adds.

4. A telescopic with a reading cap will provide a greater working distance, but a much narrower field, than a microscopic of the same magnification. Since accommodation is essentially ineffective through a telescopic, calculations of the near add are the same in practice for presbyopes and non-presbyopes.

5. The testing is carried out, as with the microscope, to determine the smallest print that can be read with the lowest magnification. Because anything viewed through a telescope appears closer than its real position, special care must be exercised to assist the patient in taking hold of the material and maintaining it at the proper distance.

6. Binocular near telescopic testing requires special arrangements for precise decentration, vertical alignment, and *convergence* of the tubes.

G. Non-spectacle aids

When the amount of magnification required for near vision has been determined, devices other than microscopic or telescopic spectacles, which will supply approximately this amount of magnification, may be tried. In this category are: hand magnifiers, stand magnifiers, clip-on telescopic magnifiers, and binocular and monocular loupes. In testing with these devices, the ease with which the patient adjusts to the device and his reaction to it should be noted.

The practitioner should familiarize himself with the various aids before having the patient try them. Some stands are adjustable but most are fixed and accommodation may or may not be required. Some of the higher power aids have better optical characteristics when used away from the eye, some closer to the eye, etc.

H. Binocularity

In testing near vision, the better eye is tested first and then the other eye. If it is found that with the same magnification there is usable vision in the two eyes, binocular prescriptions should be considered. These are only feasible in the lower orders of magnification but, when possible, they do have great utility.

If binocular prescriptions are to be considered, the fusion ability should be tested at the proposed working distance. A cover test will reveal the condition of phorias and the qualitative ability to regain fusion when it has been interrupted. Kuhns' "near vision screener" is an excellent target for this purpose.

Evaluation of fusion ability can be made, even with low visual acuities, by testing fusion with a light and a red glass or with the Worth Dot Test. A quantitative determination can be made of the ability to recover single binocular vision when loose prisms are inserted and removed.

For "weaker" adds of the order of +10.00 D., fusion may be possible with the aid of base-in prisms. The amount of prism necessary may be determined from the fusion tests described.

Where a binocular prescription is not feasible, the interference of the poorer eye may become a problem and consideration of the need to occlude it or blur it should be made.

As previously discussed, because of field losses and the location of scotomas, the eye which exhibits the best distance acuity may not be the preferred eye for reading. Where field impairments exist, a patient may find it easier to use the right eye with an $8\times$ magnification than to read with the left eye even though a $4\times$ magnification would permit the same size type to be seen. This should be kept in mind to avoid neglecting the more useful eye, because its visual acuity is much poorer.

Office Visits

When a prescription of a low vision aid is expected to ensue, it is generally best that the examination be conducted in more than one visit. The number of tests may be tiring, and often the patient's reactions are different on a second occasion. Since the attitudes and psychology of the patient form a very important part of the treatment, it is best that the doctor and the patient have a chance to become better acquainted with each other.

It is often desirable to give the patient a few ideas to think about between the first and second visits and then obtain his reactions to these suggestions. Often a patient will return with a new goal that he desires to achieve with his aids or will report that his original goal is not as important as he had previously stated.

In order to encourage the patient, and to answer his questions, it is desirable to accomplish enough during the first visit to show that vision can be improved, even though the final prescriptions have not been determined.

It is often desirable at the end of the first examination to indicate the appearance of the finished devices. Models of telescopic and microscopic lenses mounted in spectacle frames should be available. Non-spectacle devices used for testing serve as their own models. The patient may have a very false impression of the appearance of the finished device and his reaction to the true appearance of the devices should be ascertained. This will also help the patient, between visits, in considering whether or not he would want to use a device of this nature.

The patient may also have a false impression of the true size of the print that he has been reading, since it appeared so large through the testing devices. Therefore, it is advisable that he view the same test type with his previous correction.

At the second and subsequent visits some of the original findings can be rechecked. Frequently, a different magnification will be found to yield the smallest print readability or the patient may perform better or worse, *in toto*, than during the original visit. This variability should be noted and, if possible, its cause determined.

If more than one aid or type of aid will meet the same need, a comparison of their advantages and disadvantages should be made and the patient permitted to observe them himself. Describing to the patient the working distance with a microscopic as compared to a telescopic device, or the field of view with each, is not as meaningful or convincing to him as allowing him to *experience* the differences.

Chapter 8

Prescribing and Counselling

Factors Determining Success

Attitudes

The patient's attitudes should be the most important factor in determining the choice of therapies, but, too often, the practitioner's biases take precedence. Flexibility and readiness to adapt to new and diverse circumstances are desirable traits for *both* doctor and patient.

A. The doctor

Some practitioners *never* prescribe adds greater than +3.00 D.; some *never* prescribe telescopics; some prescribe *only* hand-held or stand devices; others prescribe *only* head-borne devices. Generally, those practitioners obtaining the best results for their patients seem to be the ones holding few preconceived notions restricting the choice of aids they will prescribe. Practitioners, using the eclectic and pragmatic approaches, prescribe *whatever works for this specific patient.*

B. The patient

Generally "hardening of the attitudes" accompanies hardening of the arteries and unfortunately, the majority of low vision patients are in the older age groups. Young people, usually, are more able and ready to adapt to changes such as shortened working distances and restricted fields of view, but they may be just as concerned about appearances and the opinions of others as are their seniors.

Often, one's ability to help a patient is severely restricted by other rigid stipulations, such as, insistence that one pair of spectacles must do everything, or that the aid must not be hand held. Usually, these limitations occur in combinations, which further complicates arriving at an acceptable prescription.

Flexibility may be greatly affected, at any age, by the motivation to achieve some specific goal.

Specific and Limited Goals

In determining the prescriptions, major emphasis must be placed on an analysis of the patient's specific task handicap. In simple terms, the real question is *"What does the patient want to do, visually, that he is unable to do now?"* Although this question appears simple, the answers are most important in predicting the examiner's ability to satisfy the patient's needs. *It is imperative that the patient have specific activities in mind.* Except for routine correction of refractive errors, low vision care is rarely successful if the aid is prescribed, or advice given to help the patient "to see better".

The practitioner must first analyze the patient's goals in terms of their reality in light of his handicap. If any of the patient's goals are unrealistic, they must be discussed with the patient so that he does not accept an aid with over optimistic expectations of the benefits he will derive. For example, one cannot expect a patient with 20/400 best corrected acuity will be able to drive a car using a telescopic aid. If driving a car is the only goal that this patient has, it is unlikely that he will be successful with any aid, even though it may enable him to read a newspaper or a Snellen Chart.

The prescription must be based upon that which is important to the patient, rather than that which is important to the practitioner. This does not mean that the practitioner should not discuss and demonstrate the patient's visual possibilities using aids, but the prescription must be *finally* based on the patient's motivation to attain a specific performance goal.

In arriving at the patient's true goals, some degree of caution must be exercised. Many patients do not say what they really mean. Since, in many peoples' minds reading is symbolic of the way they used to see, a patient may say he "wants to be able to read" while in reality he actually wants to be able to recognize friends down the street.

Therefore, before prescribing, it is important that a patient recognize the limitations of an aid as well as its benefits.

Motivation

Patient motivation is the *sine qua non* of success. A highly motivated patient will accept and use any reasonable prescription, making practical use of even a minimal amount of vision. Conversely, *without* adequate motivation, even a seemingly miraculous prescription will have little chance of being used successfully.

It is better to postpone prescribing until motivation is developed, even if for months or years, rather than risk an immediate failure which may discourage any future utilization of aids. Motivation has been discussed in greater detail in Chapter III, Psychological and Sociological Factors.

The Prescription

General

A general rule to be used in determining the final form of the aids is that every possible effort must be made to eliminate factors which may act as a deterrent to the patient accepting and using the aid. Very often, one must reach a compromise between optimum optics and appearance. The aid utilizing the best possible optics is of no value if the patient will not use it because of the poor appearance, weight, discomfort, or inconvenience. The relative importance of each factor differs for each patient, thus, there is no single aid which is optimum for all patients.

Economic Factors

Economics should not be an early factor in determining the prescription. The practitioner should first arrive at the optimum prescription considering all other factors. Then, if cost is an insoluble problem, less expensive devices can be considered. It is far costlier to prescribe an inexpensive, cosmetically unacceptable device, which is *not* used, than a more costly device, which the patient *does* use.

Optical Factors

A. Correction of ametropia

1. The refractive error and the effect of its correction on visual acuity and performance have been determined during the examination. Studies by the Industrial Home for the Blind (1957) and Rosenbloom (1966) have shown that a large percentage of low vision patients benefitted from ordinary spectacles to correct their ametropia.

2. The ametropia should be corrected when an improvement in visual acuity of one line is consistently demonstrated, and the patient reports that his general vision is improved. Since the many limitations of magnification devices are not inherent in the usual spectacle corrections, the latter may be prescribed more freely.

3. When prescribing a telescopic, it is generally found that cylindrical corrections of 0.50 D. or less may be omitted. However, *any* spherical or cylindrical correction which affords a recognizable improvement should be incorporated in the eyepiece of the system.

4. When prescribing a microscopic, it is generally found that cylindrical corrections of 2.00 D. or less may be omitted. However, if the cylindrical correction affords a recognizable improvement it should be incorporated. Spherical ametropic corrections may easily be considered as part of the total lens power of the microscopic. However, despite the laboratory's designation of the lens, the magnification obtained by the patient can only be calculated after the spherical ametropic correction has been subtracted algebraically from the total dioptric power.

5. An insert system consists of a carrier lens and telescopic and/or microscopic section(s). The considerations discussed in 2, 3, and 4 above apply and must be considered for each part separately.

B. Magnification

1. It is generally best to prescribe the lowest magnification which allows the patient to perform his specific tasks with a slight reserve, e.g. if the task requires reading 7 point sentences, the aid should permit the reading of 5 point sentences. A greater magnification which permits reading the 5 point with greater ease is probably unnecessary.

2. For a table of equivalent type sizes, refer to Figure V-2. Because of differences in type form, contrast, spacing, and paper quality, acuity ratings should only be thought of as approximations.

C. Working distance and working space

1. As used here *working distance* refers to the distance between the object of regard and the standard spectacle plane, while *working space* refers to the unobstructed distance between the true object and the front of the aid.

2. The working distance of a telescopic with a near add is greater than the working distance of an equivalent magnification microscopic (see Figure VIII-1A, C, D).

3. In the case of projection magnifiers, the object of regard (screen) is not the true object (see

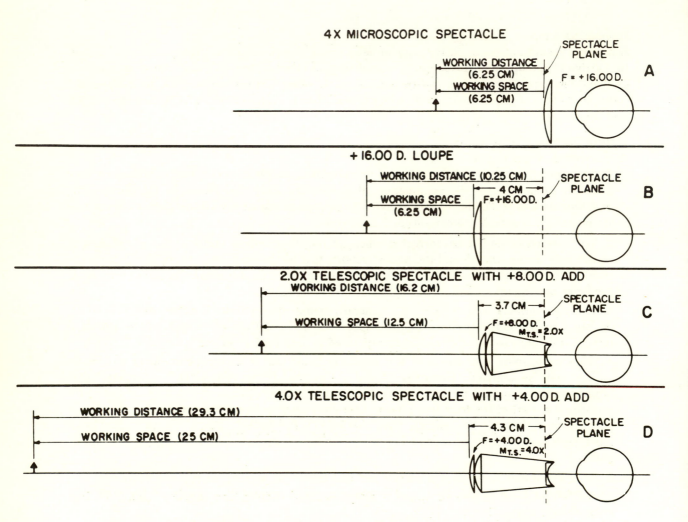

Fig. VIII-1. *Working distance and working space. In all illustrations shown, the object is in the primary focal plane of the first convex lens. All systems shown produce 4X effective magnification relative to 25cm.*

    A.   4X microscopic spectacle.
    B.   4X loupe (hand, stand, or headborne).
    C.   4X telemicroscope (2.0X telescope with a 2X add).
    D.   4X telemicroscope (4.0X telescope with a 1X add).

    Only in the case of the microscopic spectacle (A) are working distance and working space equal. In the other cases, the distance between the first convex lens and the spectacle plane must be added to the working space to equal the working distance. The important point to note here is that with the same effective magnification, the working distance and working space can be varied depending on the type of system used and its parimeters.

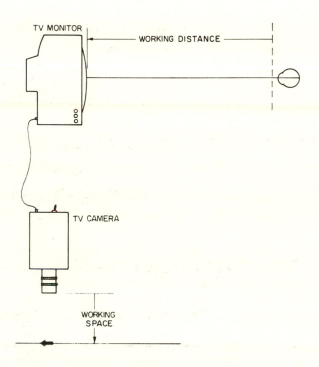

TV MONITOR

WORKING DISTANCE

TV CAMERA

WORKING
SPACE

VIII-2.   Working distance and working space for a projection magnifier (CCTV). Projection magnifiers offer the opportunity for large working distances even with high magnification. Electronic projection magnifiers (CCTV) also offer ample working space while optical projection magnifiers offer no useable working space.

Figure VIII-2). Thus, working space is independent of the working distance, unlike the lens systems illustrated in Figure VIII-1.

4. In essentially visual tasks (i.e. reading, broadcast T.V.), the *working distance* is of prime importance. In tasks involving manipulation of equipment, the *working space* is usually more important. Thus, in writing, a working space is required for the hand and pencil.

5. Patients often require multiple aids in order to provide differing working distances and working spaces with the magnifications needed for different tasks.

D. Field of view

1. Restriction of the field of view is characteristic of magnification devices.

2. Generally, as the magnification increases, the field decreases.

3. Restriction with a microscopic is much less than with a telescopic of equivalent magnification.

4. The maximum field is obtained when the aid is as close to the eye as possible, and decreases as it is moved away.

5. For the same type of device, larger diameter lenses provide a larger useful field if aberrations do not intervene.

6. Where the optical field restriction is no greater than the restriction already imposed by pathology, the size of the optical field is not a disadvantage.

7. Examples of field requirements

a. Ideally, to read a newspaper article the field should encompass at least one column width. Reading is still possible with less; however, when the field is less than one word wide, it becomes extremely difficult.

b. Reading music calls for a field large enough to include both the treble and bass staffs.

c. Reading a newspaper requires a combination of field widths. Large headlines and photographs require a larger field (and fortunately less magnification) than the regular newsprint.

d. In mobility (walking, driving, etc.) the extent of the visual field is more important than the recognition of detail. Hence, uninterrupted magnification (full-field telescopic spectacle) is contraindicated.

8. When the field requirements of a specific task have been determined, the previously mentioned factors are manipulated in arriving at the specific devices. Where multiple field requirements exist, multiple devices may be needed. Sometimes a single task must be divided into smaller components with more uniform field requirements, e.g.. if a 6 × microscopic spectacle is needed to read newsprint, a 2½ × M.S. may be supplied for scanning and headlines.

E. Telescopic parallax

1. Since an impression of foreshortened distances occurs when viewing objects through a telescope, one must consider carefully the needs for exact distance judgments during the task. This factor also makes mobility with a full-field T.S. extremely difficult.

2. In situations where distortion of perception of distances is likely to be a serious handicap, one may prescribe an insert type T.S. or a hand-held or flip-up telescope or be prepared to strenuously train the patient to compensate for the parallax. Where it will fill the need, a non-telescopic device may be a better solution.

F. Effectivity of accommodation

1. As discussed in Chapter VI - Optics, telescopics require much more accommodation than that indicated by the fixation distance. Hence it may be necessary in some instances to prescribe a focusing telescope or multiple caps (adds) for varying distances.

G. Aberrations

1. A low vision patient may not react to lens aberrations in the same way as a person with normal acuity. Thus, a more optically perfect device may not afford any added benefits to the patient and, therefore may not justify the added expense, poorer appearance, increased waiting time, etc.

2. The comparison is best made subjectively by the patient using various devices of the same magnification.

a. e.g. a patient requiring a 4× M.S. should be tested with a + 16.00 D. trial set lens, a 4× doublet, a 4× aspheric, and a 4× one piece bifocal microscopic. One patient will demonstrate an increased performance with one device, another with a different one. The authors do not know of any infallible system of predicting which aid will be judged best by the patient.

Facility, Speed, and Tolerance

In evaluating the suitability of an aid for the performance of specific tasks, it is necessary to judge more than the size of objects which can be resolved. If the task involves reading, writing, drawing, sewing, etc., the facility with which the task can be accomplished must be taken into account. The speed and the time that the patient can tolerate performing the task are also critical factors to consider. Mehr et al.(1973) found tolerance time one of the most significant factors in deciding whether to prescribe an optical aid or a closed circuit TV magnifier. Generally, reading duration time was two and one-half times greater with the CCTV than with optical aids.

Appearance Factors

A. General

1. *Before ordering any device, the practitioner should be sure that the patient knows the appearance of the finished aid.* The most positive way of accomplishing this is to have finished sample devices available for the patient to see. Attempts to describe the appearance of aids to patients or the use of photographs are generally inadequate.

2. In the case of custom devices, it is possible to obtain demonstration devices mounted into frames from the suppliers. Ready-made aids may already be available among the testing equipment. When they are not, prototypes should be obtained for the patient's inspection before a final decision is made.

B. Form of the Aid

1. Generally the more closely a device resembles ordinary spectacles, the more readily it will be accepted.

2. *From the appearance standpoint alone,* a head-borne sports binocular is less acceptable than a prescription type full field telescopic. A full field telescopic is less acceptable than an insert type telescopic. The insert telescopic in turn is less acceptable than the modern prescription type microscopics (see Figure VIII-3).

3. Press-on Fresnel lenses or prisms can be used to significantly reduce thickness. However, since all presently available Fresnel designs cause reduction in contrast, they are often poorly tolerated by many low vision patients.

4. A more detailed discussion of factors affecting appearance of spectacle aids appears in Chapter XI—Fitting, Ordering, Verifying And Dispensing.

Comfort Factors

In some instances the patient's anatomical or dermatological characteristics will require special consideration. As in the case of aphakics, one must consider whether the weight-bearing surfaces of the face will be adequate to support a heavy aid and maintain its alignment. Comfort is discussed further in Chapter XI—Fitting, Ordering, Verifying, and Dispensing.

Physical Handicaps

Since a person with one handicap often exhibits others concurrently, the low vision patient will frequently require special consideration of his other problems, e.g. when a hand tremor is present, not only is a hand held contraindicated, but a reading stand may be necessary in addition to an optical aid.

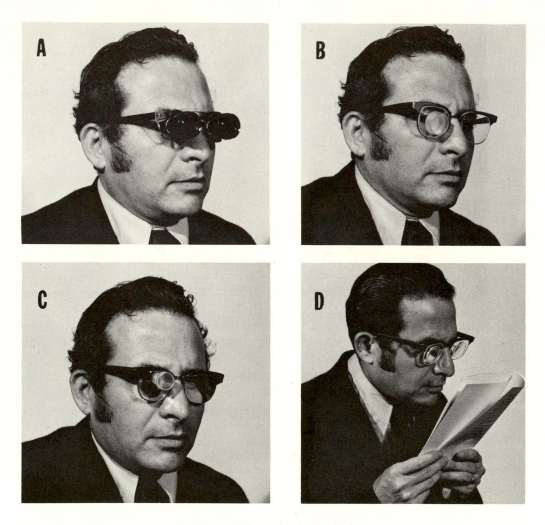

Fig. VIII-3.   Cosmesis of spectacle aids.
    A.   *Headborne sports binocular.*
    B.   *Full field telescopic spectacle.*
    C.   *Insert type telescopic spectacle.*
    D.   *Full field microscopic spectacle.*

Illumination

Having determined during the examination the optimum illumination for a specific patient to perform a particular task, the practitioner must prescribe the controls which will meet the requirements. It is not sufficient to furnish broad guidelines, but rather the practitioner should demonstrate the use of the recommended devices, lamps, visors, etc. Further, the doctor should either provide the needed control devices from his office, or relate detailed instructions and specifications for obtaining them.

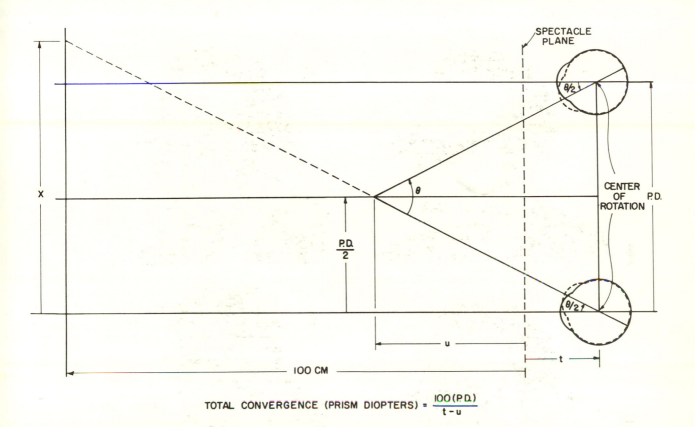

$$\text{TOTAL CONVERGENCE (PRISM DIOPTERS)} = \frac{100\,(\text{P.D.})}{t - u}$$

Fig. VIII-4.   Diagram showing total convergence required for viewing near objects and its relationship to interpupillary distance, and distance from the spectacle plane to the center of rotation of the eye. The P.D., t, and u must all be measured in the same units.

The Other Eye

A. General

Because of a multiplicity of factors, few low vision patients are capable of achieving single binocular vision. The low vision aids themselves often preclude binocularity.

Most authorities agree that the practical limit for binocular microscopics is approximately +10.00 D. (Thus 2½×).

Binocular telescopics for near vision are made in powers up to 5×, but are rarely used in powers above 3.5×.

For hand held and stand magnifiers, binocular use is limited by the interdependent factors of lens diameter, aberrations, and eye to lens distance. Large diameter magnifiers which can be used binocularly are all of relatively low power.

Projection magnifiers do permit large amounts of magnification with working distances long enough for comfortable, single, binocular vision.

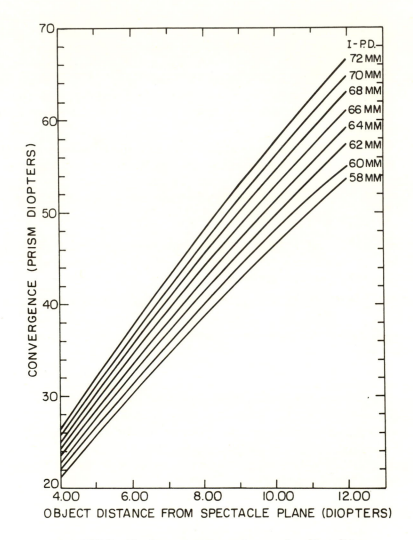

Fig. VIII-5.   Total convergence requirement for object distances of 25cm. to 8.3cm. for various interpupillary distances. The spectacle plane was assumed to be 2.5cm. from the center of rotation of the eye.

B. Binocularity
    1. Although its achievement creates problems, binocular vision also has advantages.
        a. Scotomas in the field of one eye may not be exactly duplicated in the other, thus affording a binocular field more complete than that of either eye separately.
        b. Visual acuity may be better and more stable.
        c. A wider field is available.
        d. Psychologically, patients feel happier using both eyes.
    2. Binocularity requires equal magnification for the two eyes. The magnification should be that which is required by the eye which performs the specific task better.

3. Binocular use of strong adds entails such large amounts of convergence that base-in prism is invariably required (see Figure VIII-4).

For the amounts of decentration required for the near interpupillary distances *alone*, see Figure XI-1, Chapter XI; however, additional amounts of base-in prism are required to facilitate fusion. Figure VIII-5 shows the *total* amounts of convergence required for object distances between 25 and 8.3 cm. The amount of prism prescribed depends on many factors (distance, heterophoria, fusional reserves and quality, etc.), hence is usually less than the total convergence requirement.

4. If telescopics are to be used binocularly at near distances, the tubes must be angled to meet in the fixation plane. Since this angle varies for different fixation distances, a given telescopic system can only be used binocularly at one distance unless the angle between the tubes is adjustable. A telescopic system set for binocularity at one distance may be used monocularly at another distance by changing one add and occluding the other eye.

C. Monocularity

1. If the other eye has no useful vision, a balance lens may be prescribed. Many patients will prefer that the balance lens resemble the working lens, even though greater expense is involved, and the patient should be given this option.

2. One may prescribe a reversible frame with different devices or powers in the two sides for flexibility.

3. In those instances where the poorer eye interferes with the better seeing one, an occluder should be considered.

D. Bi-ocularity

1. If both eyes have useful vision, but single binocular vision is not attainable or desirable, one may prescribe differently for the two eyes allowing greater flexibility, e.g. an 8× M.S. (+32.00 D.) might be prescribed for one eye to read fine newsprint while a 2× M.S. (+8.00 D.) in bifocal form might be prescribed for the other eye to scan the headlines, to afford working space for writing, and to permit some distance vision.

2. Feasibility of bi-ocular prescriptions cannot be determined on a strictly theoretical basis but should be subjected to a performance test.

Commonplace Needs

A. In the past, great emphasis in low vision care has been placed upon improving the patient's ability to read Snellen charts and newsprint using some type of spectacles. Unfortunately many of the requirements of everyday living have been neglected.

B. Because low vision aids are restricting, when a device is prescribed for a specific task, it will seldom also satisfy the majority of other daily visual needs. Hence, to meet these needs, multiple aids are required.

1. A presbyopic patient who has a microscopic spectacle with a very short working distance and a narrow field will still have difficulties writing, eating, cooking, locating an article in the newspaper, or finding a bill in a file. To perform these types of tasks an "intermediate" add (approximately one-third the microscopic add, but usually not more than +10.00 D.), must be provided, probably in multifocal form. Very often partially-sighted patients carry a variety of folding magnifiers in different powers.

2. Many patients require magnification for everyday distance vision greater than that available in telescopic spectacles. Compact hand held telescopes up to 10× are obtainable and useful

for such tasks as: reading street signs, house numbers, chalkboards, score boards, etc. Genensky (1973) advocates the use of binoculars for these purposes, even for people having only monocular vision.

3. For shaving, applying make-up, combing hair, etc., magnifying mirrors may be useful.

4. Many special, non-optical devices are available which can be extremely helpful for everyday tasks (see Chapter XV—Non-optical Aids).

Management of the Poor Prognosis Patient

General

A. In those cases in which the factors pointing towards success are not present, the practitioner should not attempt to convince the patient to accept an aid to justify the time and money already spent on evaluation procedures. Practitioners should realize that some patients receive great benefit from the examination procedures and counseling alone.

1. Some patients will never accept an aid, but need to be reassured from time to time that they are not "blind", or that there has been no further loss of vision.

2. There are also those patients whose self-image is improved by the examination procedures alone. The patient who undergoes a low vision analysis because he "cannot read a newspaper," but then refuses to accept a proposed aid because he "does not want to hold the newspaper *that* close" or "will not wear anything that looks like *that*" has still received some benefit. When he came for the examination he thought his vision so poor that he *could not* read. After the examination he realized he *could* read but did not *choose* to do so. The difference between these two attitudes may seem slight to the normally sighted, but to the partially-sighted, there is a difference significant enough with some patients to alter their entire psychological attitude and thus their everyday activities. The patient may no longer think of himself as a blind person.

B. It is helpful to have a responsible third party accompany the patient during the examination, demonstrations and discussions. Then later if the patient complains of his inability to perform a desired task, this witness may be able to remind the patient that he *could* perform that task if he had obtained the aid that he used in the doctor's office.

The Rejecting Patient

A. Patients refuse to accept aids for a number of reasons such as recency, dependence, pride, vanity, etc. See Chapter III—Psychological and Sociological Factors.

B. Some simple instructions, for example, concerning illumination, may be accepted.

C. The further course of action depends upon the cause of the rejection.

1. In cases of recency, pride, and vanity the practitioner should advise the patient (and third party) of the present possibilities of help from low vision aids while acknowledging the patient's stated objections and conveying that the patient's feelings are understood. The patient should be instructed to return in six to twelve months since "new advances in optometric science are constantly occurring". Meanwhile, if one can communicate with the third party, he may assist in altering the patient's attitudes during the interval.

2. In dependency or other situations where some psychological need is being served by the handicap, psychotherapy must precede the prescribing of an aid.

The Dubious Prognosis

A. In those cases where performance with an aid is questionable because of factors such as senility, mental retardation, severe emotional upsets, or rapidly deteriorating vision, the prescription of aids is best limited to those which are simple, inexpensive and quickly obtainable, e.g. an inexpensive illuminated stand magnifier requires little training and may be immediately available.

B. Counseling concerning non-optical aids such as talking books, signature stencils, self-threading needles, etc. may be extremely valuable. Social counseling such as information about tax exemptions, blind benefits, rehabilitation services, etc., should be included.

The Hopeless Prognosis

A. In those few cases where it has been determined that optical aids are of no assistance, the patient may still benefit from counseling, as discussed in the preceding paragraph. In addition, the doctor should inform the patient and his family of agencies serving the visually handicapped (i.e., blind centers; Braille libraries; American Foundation for the Blind; American Printing House for the Blind; etc.) and of services such as mobility training, daily living skills training, tapes and recordings for the blind; reader services, etc.

B. Koetting (1962) suggests that all low vision patients should receive four specific suggestions and further states, "No matter how hopeless the case may seem, we never had an occasion when we could not think of four specific suggestions."

General Comments

Counseling

A. While counseling has already been discussed in relation to management of the Poor Prognosis Patient, all low vision patients benefit from proper counseling.

   1. Any practitioner who plans to care for partially-sighted patients, himself, should become acquainted with non-optical aids and how the patient can obtain them (see Chapter XV—Non-Optical Aids).

   2. Similarly, he should become acquainted with laws, regulations, agencies, organizations, and other community facilities relating to the totally and partially-blind so that he might advise his patients concerning social services and legal benefits.

   3. Counseling should also include educational and vocational components.

      a. Not only should the patient be counseled, but often information must be transmitted to relatives, guardians, teachers, employers, rehabilitation counselors, etc.

      b. Reports should be in simple language rather than technical jargon and should include the basic information on the patient's visual capabilities and limitations which is needed by the recipient in making decisions for the patient's welfare.

B. The Team Approach

Ideally, management of the low vision patient involves many disciplines. Best results are obtained when they work cooperatively and keep each other informed. This is most easily achieved within the framework of an agency but can be accomplished for private patients by referral and communication. Members of the team, in addition to the optometrist or ophthalmologist interested in low vision, can include:

   1. Educators, including regular classroom teachers and teachers of the visually handicapped, school administrators, school psychologists and school nurses

2. Social agency workers, including medical social workers, eligibility counselors and Aid to Blind social workers

3. Rehabilitation counselors, including vocational rehabilitation counselors, home teachers for visually impaired adults and counselors at sheltered workshops and orientation centers

4. Psychological counselors, including psychologists, psychiatrists and psychiatric social workers

5. Orientation and mobility instructors, also known as peripatologists

6. Health care workers, including all medical practitioners, other ophthalmologists, other optometrists, public health nurses, administrators and nurses in rest homes, nursing homes and rehabilitation hospitals

7. Low vision instructors, including optometric aides and optical aids counselors

8. Librarians, including those working primarily with the handicapped.

Evaluation

A. By the doctor

1. In arriving at the final form of the prescription(s) the practitioner must consider all of the previously discussed factors, pitting one against the other in light of the patient's needs and desires until the best compromise is attained.

B. With the patient

1. After arriving at the final prescription, it is wise to discuss with the patient the advantages versus the exact limitations of the particular device. The patient will then know, when the device is finally dispensed, what he *will* and *will not* be able to do with the aid.

2. This is the time for the practitioner to answer questions and to consider revisions of the prescription in view of the patient's comments.

Programming

A. Because of the need in many instances of multiple prescriptions and because of the complexity of some devices, aids may be programmed over a period of time.

1. Programming allows the patient to concentrate on learning to use one or two devices at a time.

2. It also allows the patient to discover for himself those visual tasks which still present great difficulties. Thus, the need for multiple aids to solve multiple problems becomes apparent to the patient as well as the doctor.

B. Periodic re-evaluations are even more essential for the partially-sighted than for the more routine patient.

1. Where the perception of detail has been curtailed for some time or never developed, it often is found that this ability improves with use and consequently a lower power aid may suffice.

2. Where old pathology progresses or new pathology occurs, further deterioration of vision may require a higher power aid.

3. New demands (as in growing children) may require different solutions.

Prescription Axioms

A. THE PATIENT MUST HAVE *AT LEAST ONE SPECIFIC TASK* IN MIND. (See Chapter VII—The Low Vision Examination.)

B. THE PATIENT MUST BE ABLE TO ACCOMPLISH *THE SPECIFIC TASK* BETTER WITH THE AID THAN WITHOUT IT.

C. THE PATIENT *MUST KNOW* HOW THE *FINISHED* AID WILL LOOK *BEFORE* IT IS ORDERED.

D. THE PATIENT MUST *DEMONSTRATE PROFICIENCY* IN USING THE AID IN THE OFFICE *BEFORE* TAKING IT HOME. (See Chapter XIII—Training.)

Chapter 9

Control of Illumination

Introduction

Most people with low vision experience problems with illumination. They may require high, medium or low levels of illumination, be very sensitive to glare and contrast and require unusually long periods for photopic or scotopic adaptations.

The patient who has suffered an adventitious vision loss later in life may persist in using illumination levels more appropriate to his previous better vision. Some people continue to follow the advice of an earlier authority long after the circumstances have changed. Others have habitually adapted to the environment and do not readily think in terms of adapting the environment to their needs.

With some patients, control of illumination is the most helpful and sometimes sole prescription required. With most patients, magnification and illumination control are *both* required.

General Considerations

The Inverse Square Law

$$\text{Illuminance} = \frac{\text{candle power of source}}{(\text{source to surface distance})^2}$$

This is not well understood by the general public who tend to think of illumination mainly in terms of the brightness of the source and, for example, realize that doubling the power of the light source doubles the illuminance. They do not realize that halving the distance between the same source and the illuminated surface would quadruple the illuminance (see Figure IX-1).

The Cosine Law

The illuminance varies with the cosine of the angle between the source and the perpendicular to the surface (see Figure IX-2).

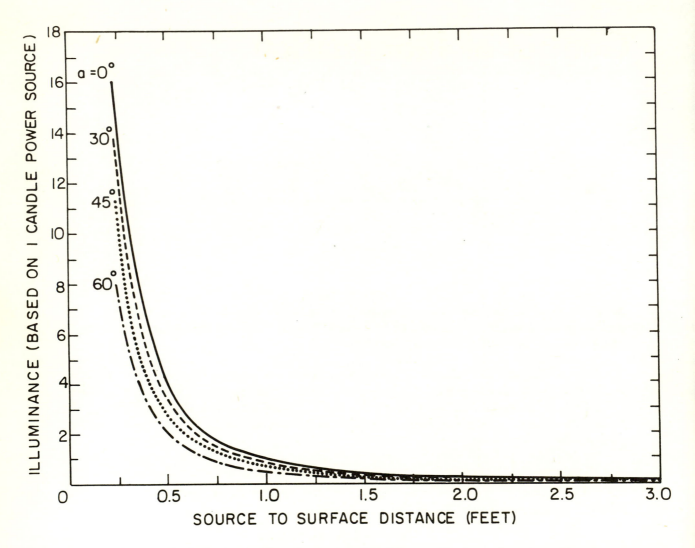

Fig. IX-1. *Graph showing the effect of source to surface distance on illuminance for various source angles.*

The Inverse Square Law and Cosine Law can be combined into the formula:

$$\text{Illuminance} = \frac{\text{cosine angle a (candle power source)}}{(\text{source to surface distance})^2}$$

The greatest effect is thus produced when the source is perpendicular to the surface (see Figure IX-1).

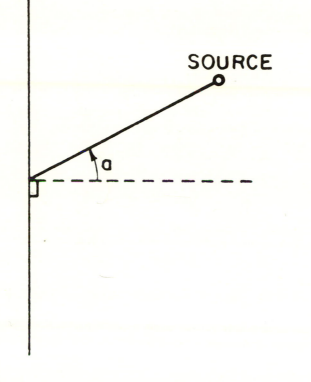

Fig. IX-2.   Diagram defining angle a for The Cosine Law.

Reflectance
The reflectance of the surface must be considered. Glossy magazines present a different problem than dull newsprint.

Physiological Optics
The effect of illumination on the retina, pupil, and the refracting media all need to be considered.

Etiological Considerations

The Optic Nerve and Retina
A. *Senile macular degeneration; macular holes; diabetic retinopathy; old central chorioretinitis; optic atrophy; glaucoma; coloboma of the retina, choroid, and optic nerve; and degenerative myopia* generally require high levels of illumination.

B. *Retinitis Pigmentosa*

1. Poor dark adaptation is an early and persistent characteristic.

2. High levels of illumination are generally required.

3. Posterior subcapsular cataract is a frequent complication and may require elimination of all extraneous light.

C. *Albinism* (which also involves hypopigmentation of other structures)
   1. Albinos are generally sensitive to bright light.
   2. Extraneous light should be eliminated when possible.
D. *Achromatopsia*
   1. Rod achromats do not tolerate high levels of illumination well.
   2. These patients experience great difficulty with changes in the level of illumination.
   3. Low levels of illumination and elimination of extraneous light are helpful.
   4. Absorptive filters transmitting principally red light are sometimes useful.
E. *Retrobulbar neuritis and some severe macular degenerations* may require lower levels of illumination.

The Crystalline Lens
A. *Cataracts*
   1. Central opacities cause more problems with a small pupil, hence require reduced light or mydriatic drugs.
   2. Many opacities become luminous sources setting up a veiling glare, hence require minimal extraneous light incident on the eye.
   3. Opacities absorb and scatter light so that higher levels of illumination are required to penetrate to the retina.
   4. Due to increased crystalline lens fluorescence from violet and ultra-violet, incandescent sources may be preferable to fluorescent sources.
B. *Aphakia*
   1. Aphakes may require decreased illumination.
   2. Ultra-violet absorption is indicated.

The Iris
A. *Aniridia* may require lower levels of illumination, but often it is not a great problem.
B. *Pinpoint pupils* require high levels of illumination.

The Cornea
A. *Central opacities* may permit better vision with a larger pupil accomplished by reducing the light incident on the eye or by mydriatic drugs.
B. *Keratoconus* may require increased illumination.
C. *Multiple opacities, or corneal dystrophy*
   1. These conditions may require increased illumination to penetrate the opacities.
   2. Opacities may become luminous sources and hence require elimination of extraneous light.

Age
Due to a combination of factors affecting various structures of the eye Guth (1957) found older people required twice the illumination of a younger group. Since so many low vision patients are over 60 this is significant. It also means that the same special care of illumination which is helpful to persons with reduced acuity will also be helpful for older persons with normal acuity.

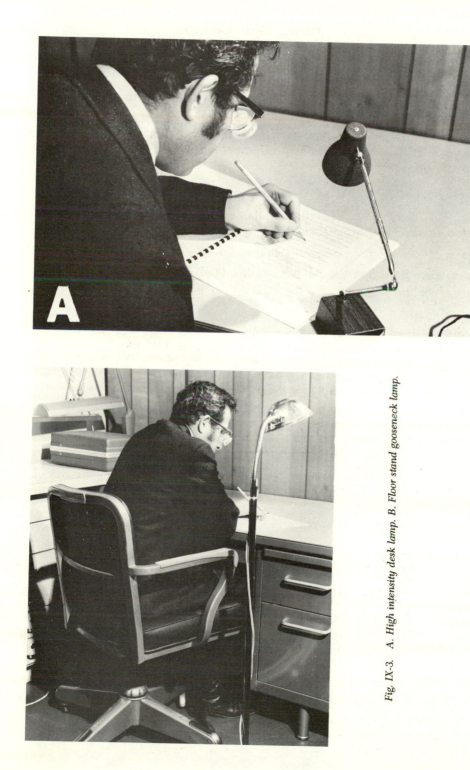

Fig. IX-3.   A. High intensity desk lamp. B. Floor stand gooseneck lamp.

Illumination Controls

Lamps

A. High levels of illumination can be obtained inexpensively by markedly reducing the distance from the source.

B. Where the lamp may be in front of the patient it is important that the shade be completely opaque.

C. Small high intensity lamps work very well for the patient who requires high levels of illumination. A floor stand gooseneck lamp may be the choice for reading or sewing while seated in a large chair (see Figure IX-3).

The Typoscope

A. Prentice (1897) described a non-reflecting dull black shield with a slit in it to be placed over the page. It still remains an extremely useful device for eliminating extraneous light.

B. There are a couple of typoscopes available commercially (see Figures VII-12 and XIV-67).

C. Custom sizes can be made from dull black railroad board (obtainable at stationers).

    1. Morgan (1962) has suggested that the ideal slit size is 3 lines high by 1 column wide.

Visors

Elimination of overhead light may be very helpful.

A. Visors that fit on spectacle frames are available (see Figure XIV-68).

B. Hat brims are useful.

C. The "tennis visor" is an alternative for the non-spectacle wearer.

Side Shields

A. Where obstruction of peripheral vision will not cause a problem, opaque side shields can be used.

B. Side shields can clip on or be permanently attached to spectacles (see Figure XIV-71).

Lens Tints and Color Coatings

These can be used where specific or uniform absorption of wavelengths is indicated.

Stenopaic Slits and Holes

A. Devices of this type can be used where illumination control is indicated (see Figure XIV-71).

B. Generally, mobility is restricted with these devices.

Testing

The efficacy of illumination controls can only be correctly evaluated when the appropriate illumination environment exists or is simulated.

Policoff (1968) has pointed out that many patients who reject pinhole spectacles in an examining room will eagerly accept them if the test situation is transferred outdoors in the sunlight.

Chapter 10

Helping the Patient with a Visual Field Limitation

General

Most partially-sighted patients also have some visual field loss. While magnifying devices are of great assistance in overcoming macular area losses, they are of little assistance in overcoming peripheral field losses. Although acuity may be scarcely affected, a major field loss can cause serious problems in visual functioning. The legal definition of blindness, which is based on a field of 20 degrees or less, does not cover such major problems as hemianopias or quadrantanopias.

Although a few optical aids have been devised for coping with field limitations, they are of very limited usefulness. In many instances the best the optometrist or ophthalmologist has to offer is enlightenment, advice, and training.

Defining the Problem

Observations

Careful observations of the patient's behavior, especially his mobility and head and eye movements, afford clues to visual field limitations. A person with 20/400 acuity and only central field loss will generally not bump into furniture, doorways, or cabinets. This type of behavior would point towards a peripheral field loss.

History

Reports of excessive problems in dim light, especially night blindness, are suggestive of loss of rod vision, thus a peripheral involvement. Also, reports of consistently being clumsy or bumping into things on one side or above or below suggests a field loss. Likewise, reports of skipping words or losing the place in reading may indicate a field loss.

Refractive Examination
Difficulty in locating the charts or fixation targets should arouse suspicion. Consistently omitting one area of the Snellen chart is an indicator of a field loss in the area omitted. Ability to read smaller letters when larger letters at the same distance are missed, is usually a sign of a small functional field.

Ophthalmoscopy
Retinal or optic nerve changes observed in specific areas may indicate affected areas of the field. It is also true that field changes can exist from retro-bulbar involvement without any visible changes in the fundus.

Perimetry
The definitive tests are performed with the perimeter and tangent screen. Screening tests, such as confrontation, Harrington-Flocks Multiple Pattern Screener, and the Friedman Visual Field Analyser may provide useful information towards further investigation, or indicate the area of loss when poor fixation or poor cooperation make lengthier testing impractical.

Effect on Visual Skills

Single Binocular Vision
A. Maintenance of binocular vision is hampered by large scotomas. In the absence of diplopia, fusional movements are not stimulated. Hence, a significant phoria may become an intermittent tropia.

B. Pseudo-tropias may be found on the cover test where a central scotoma causes eccentric viewing. The eyes may be in perfect orthophoric alignment until the better eye is covered. The image then falls upon a central scotoma and the eye moves to place the image upon a functional (but eccentric) area of the retina. This movement can be mistaken by the novice for a tropia.

C. Although field defects interfere with binocular vision, diplopia rarely results, since scotomas make "suppression" areas par excellence.

D. Stereopsis is diminished by central field losses and by increased binocular problems.

Awareness of Surroundings
A. Locating objects becomes difficult with a very narrow field.

B. Mobility is impaired by loss of information from the affected areas of the visual field. Bumping into objects, stumbling, and uncertainty result.

C. Social awkwardness becomes a problem. Friends passing and waving are snubbed. A hand extended to be shaken is ignored. A full glass is tipped over.

D. Working around moving machinery and driving automobiles or airplanes becomes hazardous.

Reading and Writing
Management of the written language can become a confusing problem for a person with certain types of field loss.

A. A scotoma to the right of fixation causes the next word in the line of print to disappear and is very confusing when trying to read (see Figure IV-5).

B. A right hemianopia, besides causing loss of the following word, also causes difficulty in judging the position of the right hand margin.

C. A left hemianopia, or a left scotoma, causes difficulty in locating the beginning of a line.

Adaptation to Changing Light Levels

A. Peripheral field loss means loss of rod vision and brings with it problems in dark adaptation and, when severe, total night blindness.

B. Massive central field loss is accompanied by loss of cone vision causing the loss of photopic vision and color vision.

Alleviating the Problem

Optical Aids

The use of optical aids for other than macular field defects has only limited success. However, if all circumstances are right and the patient is persistent and determined, some can be aided by optical means.

A. Minifiers can be used to present more information on the same area of retina. The Galilean telescope, when reversed, so that the concave lens becomes the objective and the convex lens the ocular, produces angular minification. The image on the retina, being minified, represents a greater amount of the object on a given retinal area than the non-minified image would. However, the minified image is also harder to discriminate because the detail in it subtends a smaller angle at the retina.

This type of aid is only practical when the macular field is intact but the peripheral field very limited, and while central acuity remains good. Occasionally, this situation is found with glaucoma, or retinitis pigmentosa.

A hand-held reversed telescope (usually about 2.5×) can be used for locating larger objects in a non-familiar environment.

Some success has been obtained by using a small insert reverse telescope in a carrier lens. The Model II Bioptic (Designs for Vision) can be readily adapted for this purpose.

B. Mirror hemianopia spectacles have been described by various people since Igersheimer (1919) with some variations in design. The most common is a small mirror attached nasally to the front of the spectacle frame (see Figure X-1). Accounts of variations, or rediscoveries of this device, appear periodically in the ophthalmic literature. Objects on the blind side are reflected into the seeing side of the eye (see Figure X-2). There is a mirror reversal of the image and where binocular vision exists, superimposition of images. Movement can be detected but form is more difficult.

Fitting requires time, patience, and much special effort. The patient must be willing to train and adapt. Most reports are of one or two successful patients, with more failures mentioned or ignored. Nooney (1972) reports on a pilot study in which 12 patients benefitted by using his device. Some of his patients have compared getting used to the device to learning to use the rear view mirror of an automobile.

Nooney uses a plastic mirror attached to the spectacle frame. He says that each mirror device must be constructed on an individual basis depending on patient need. Sometimes a second or third device had to be made before maximum efficiency was obtained.

Weiss (1969) describes a 45 degree half-silvered thin glass mirror which he cemented to the front

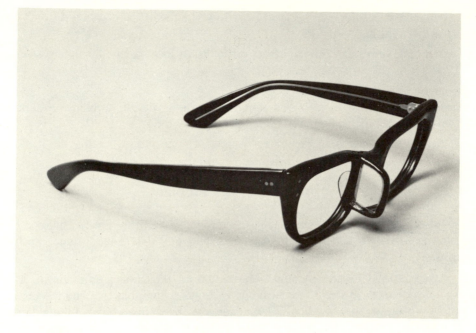

Fig. X-1.   *Mirror hemianopia spectacles.*

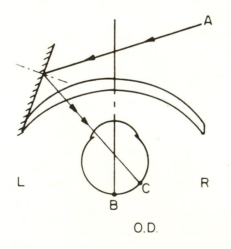

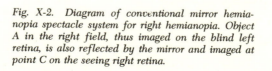

Fig. X-2.   *Diagram of conventional mirror hemianopia spectacle system for right hemianopia. Object A in the right field, thus imaged on the blind left retina, is also reflected by the mirror and imaged at point C on the seeing right retina.*

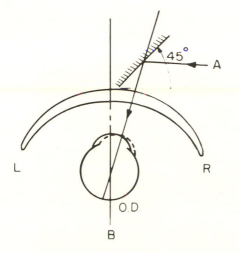

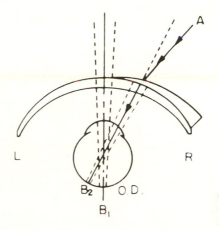

Fig. X-3. Diagram of a mirror hemianopia spectacle using a mirror attached directly to the spectacle lens for a right hemianopia, after Weiss,, 1969. Object A, in the blind field is only seen when the eye is turned to the right, however the amount the eye must be turned is much less than if object A were viewed directly. (Reproduced by permission of The Journal of the American Optometric Association).

Fig. X-4. Diagram of hemianopia spectacle using a prism attached directly to the spectacle lens for a right hemianopia, after Weiss, 1969. Object A, in the blind field is only seen when the eye is turned to the right, however, the angle through which the eye must rotate is less than if the object A were viewed directly. (Reproduced by permission of The Journal of the American Optometric Association).

surface of the lens on the temporal half, instead of to the frame at the nasal side (see Figure X-3). The main problem with this system is its fragility, he claims.

C. Partial prisms have been described by Weiss (1969, 1972). He describes the use of a 15 prism diopter prism covering the blind field (apex centrally located)(see Figure X-4). At first this was accomplished by cementing a glass prism to the surface of the lens. Later press-on Fresnel prisms were used (see Figure X-5). These can be used binocularly and on both nasal and temporal areas of the lens for small central fields such as those encountered in retinitis pigmentosa. The placement of the prisms is critical. The use of press-on vinyl prisms facilitates easy change in size and placement.

With this partial prism system, a slight eye movement brings objects located in the blind field into view. Weiss (1972) says, "The adaptation of the patient is extremely important. The initial problem is to teach the patient not to sweep his eyes from one edge of the lens to the other when walking; only one section of the lens must be used when he is moving. In the event that he wants to change his fixation he must stop walking, make the change, and then continue. On the other hand, movement of the eyes when the patient is stationary is much less of a problem and indeed, demonstrates the value of this system."

D. Projection magnifiers, both optical and electronic, are usually equipped with movable tables or scanning devices. These permit fixation on one spot on the viewing screen while the print moves across the line of vision. When scotomas make saccadic movements uncertain, this method of reading may present advantages. This seems to be particularly true for those having a large central

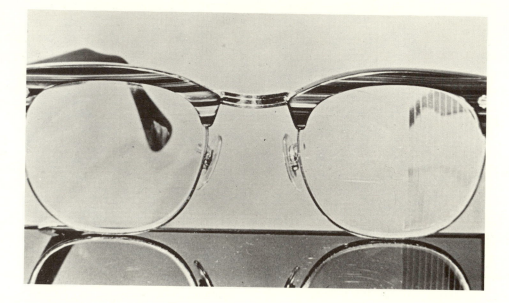

Fig. X-5. Hemianopia partial prism spectacles using a Fresnel Press-on prism for a left hemianopia of the left eye where the right eye is totally blind.

scotoma, who must use eccentric viewing and have not become well adapted to its use. Maintaining the correct angle of eccentric viewing while making saccadic movements may present problems for them. With a projection on a screen the correct eccentric fixation point is selected and can be maintained as the print moves across the screen.

Non-Optical Aids

A. Canes serve a double function in mobility for those with severe vision impairments. They can be used to inform the low vision patient about the environment he is approaching. They can also inform others that this person cannot be expected to see them. This latter is particularly valuable when crossing streets as a warning to motorists.

Many partially-sighted people who can use their vision in some circumstances but not others (e.g. in different lighting conditions) prefer to carry folding canes in their pockets or purses for use as needed.

B. Guide dogs are rarely used by the partially-sighted since they require constant care and do not lend themselves well to periodic use.

C. New technology is developing many substitutes for visual observation of the environment. Presently they are in development rather than mass production and are quite expensive. For the present, they are likely to be used mainly by the totally blind.

1. Kay (1965) Sensors are worn like hearing-aid spectacles with an earphone in each ear. They use ultrasound which is projected from the front center of the spectacle frame and picked up again by two small microphones after echoing from objects in front of the user. The ultrasound is converted to audible sound before transmission to the ears of the user.

The Doppler effect is helpful in detecting movements and the sound received from hard and soft objects varies. With practice, much information about the environment, especially at head level, can be gleaned.

2. Laser canes focus and detect a narrow laser beam at a set distance and angle. They can be used to detect steps, holes, and obstacles. The signal is converted to tactile and audible output (Benjamin, 1968).

D. Reading guides help to overcome the problem of losing words or finding the right or left hand margins. This guide can be a typoscope, 3 × 5 card, ruler, or finger. The kinesthetic sense can be used to help locate a margin and guide the visual alignment.

Counseling and Training

In many instances, the most useful assistance we can give the patient with visual field limitations is in the area of counseling and training. The counseling may be required not only for the patient, but also for family members, teachers, employers, mobility instructors, etc.

A. A tangent screen can easily become a teaching aid to show the patient and others the extent of the limitation. The limitation and its practical consequences need to be explained and understood.

B. Compensatory eye movements should be explained and practiced. The general principle is to move the eyes so as to look into the blind area. Thus a field defect to the right necessitates looking toward the right to examine the blind area with the useable visual field.

C. Eccentric viewing may be necessary with an extensive field defect. After the most advantageous eccentric viewing direction is determined, it needs to be practiced.

D. Head movements rather than eye movements should be used for a very small useable field to facilitate scanning and locating. Head movements can be slower and more certain without loss of information on areas between fixations, which occurs with saccadic eye movements.

E. Adapting the environment will facilitate ease of functioning. When the patient knows the location of the blind areas of the visual field some common sense adaptations can be made in the environment. A few examples will indicate the type of things that can be done. With an inferior field defect, furniture should not be casually moved, especially low pieces like ottomans. With a superior defect, sliding door cabinets rather than outward swinging doors are advisable. With a lateral defect, a glass of water or hot coffee should be placed on the seeing rather than the blind side.

In reading, a scotoma immediately to the right of fixation is more of a problem than one to the left. An adaptation can be made by turning the page upside down and reading from right to left or turning the page 90 degrees and reading vertically. If the scotoma is more lateral than vertical, turning the page up to 45 degrees may be easier than a full 90 or 180 degree turn. When material is being prepared that must be read back, use of larger letters and more separation between lines will help prevent confusion and loss of place on the line.

F. Orientation and mobility specialists originally worked almost exclusively with the totally blind. However, they are realizing that there is a need for their services by many partially-sighted individuals. Teaching the use of the long cane is only a part of their instruction. They also teach use of the other senses as vision substitutes. Many have integrated utilization of residual vision into their programs with the use of visual scanning patterns and training with telescopes for spotting and identification of signs and landmarks.

Mobility specialists have so much to offer that it is unwise to merely advise a person to "get a cane". A brief training course by a mobility specialist will be much more rewarding.

Chapter 11

Fitting, Ordering, Verifying and Dispensing

Fitting and Ordering

Mounting Specifications

A. General

The various factors relating to frame selection often lead to mutually exclusive specifications. In most instances a compromise is determined by the relative importance of the opposing factors.

Frame design should allow the lens system to be fitted as close to the eye as possible in order to afford the largest possible useable field.

B. Appearance

1. In most instances frame selection is dictated by factors other than appearance. The frame specifications are often decided by the special requirements of the lenses, such as a need for adjustable pads, rigidity of the bridge, maintenance of exact vertex depth, etc. Within the necessary limitations, latitude exists for cosmetic styling to improve the overall appearance.

2. In the case of non-lenticular lenses, the smaller the eye size and the less extreme the shape, the thinner the lens can be made.

3. Thick, dark frames tend to conceal edges of thick lenses as well as help to control light reflections within the lenses.

C. Eye size

1. The vertical and horizontal dimensions of the eye must be sufficient to accept the carrier in insert or multiple lens systems.

2. When using high add bifocals, aberrations, optical center position, and shortened working distance restrict the useable linear field. The shape and dimensions of the lens must allow a large segment area and permit a high placement of the resultant optical center through the segment.

D. Bridge

1. In most instances adjustable arms and pads are to be preferred; however, fixed nose pads may be used for microscopics if caution is exercised in the original centering. For telescopics, the maximum bridge adjustability and rigidity are required.

2. When using adjustable arms and pads, an extra wide bridge will allow for any needed lateral adjustment.

E. Temples

1. Temples should be sturdy enough, long enough, and of a style to hold the aid in place and retain their adjustment once set.

2. For the difficult cases, athletic head bands may be quite useful.

3. Temple-front joints must allow for radical angling where needed. In some cases, as much as 15 to 20 degrees angling is required to obtain the optimum pantoscopic angle.

F. Comfort

1. The frame should be as light as possible, consistent with the previously mentioned factors. Bearing surfaces should be as large as possible to distribute weight over a wide area.

2. Ancillary frame comfort aids, such as plastic or rubber sponge nosepad cushions, temple covers, etc., can be used when needed.

G. Positioning

Location and orientation of low vision aids is generally more critical and more important than with ordinary spectacles. Telescopics and inserts generally require more exact placement than full diameter microscopics. Thus the exact fit of the mounting should be ascertained before lens specifications are written.

Lens Specifications

A. The following aspects of lens prescription must be considered in ordering low vision aids:

1. Magnification
2. Ametropia correction
3. Form and material
4. Tint, coating, etc.
5. Centering
6. Position of various elements

B. Magnification and ametropia correction

1. In microscopic spectacles, magnification and ametropia correction may be combined and designated as total lens power. This is discussed in more detail in Chapter VIII—Prescribing and Counseling.

2. Many ready-made telescopic devices may have an ametropic correction incorporated by cementing the appropriate lens to the back of the ocular lens system or by placing the prescription lens into the proper size camera filter holder and attaching that to the ocular side of the system.

4. All specifications (sphere, cylinder, tint, coating, etc.) for insert systems should state whether they are to be incorporated throughout the system or are to be limited only to the carrier or only to the insert.

5. Ordering ready-made magnifiers, loupes, etc. poses special problems for which there are no universal solutions. In those few instances where catalogues specify magnification one has no indication of which magnification formula was used. Many times one is at a loss to know if the numerical specification relates to lens diameter, focal length, magnification, or dioptric power. Even where specifications are clear, there is no assurance that the product will match them. Reordering a known device may still be hazardous since these suppliers have a tendency to change their products without changing the catalogue specifications. The only safe system the authors have been able to devise is to dispense the device presently in hand.

C. Form and material

    1. The usual advantages and disadvantages of glass and plastic lenses apply. In addition the following must be considered:

        a. Choice of material is often restricted by the limited availability of many low vision aids.

        b. Safety

    Lenses with large differences in thickness may be more susceptible to breakage after heat tempering than before. For these lenses, chemical hardening is preferable.

        c. The use of Fresnel press-on prisms and lenses extends the range of prescription lenses which otherwise are not readily available. They are especially useful for reducing lens thickness or adding prism where it otherwise cannot be incorporated as in bifocal segments. Except for thickness considerations cementing glass or plastic lenses will accomplish the same ends.

    2. Base curves

        a. Base curves of standard series may be manipulated to some extent to afford more ideal optics for very short working distances. This is discussed further in Chapter VI—Optics.

        b. A high power convex lens appears better cosmetically if made in the biconvex form. Fonda (1965) states that for powers of +8.00 D. to +14.00 D. the ocular surface should be plano; for +16.00 D. the ocular surface should be +2.00 D.; for +20.00 D. the ocular surface should be +4.00 D.; and for +24.00 D. the ocular surface should be +8.00 D.

        c. Above +12.00 D. many low vision practitioners use aspheric lenses, reduced diameter (lenticular) lenses, or doublets and triplets.

    3. Dioptric powers of the usual single vision lenses obtained through regular ophthalmic laboratories are specified in terms of back vertex power. This fact must be considered where high power thick and/or highly curved lenses are employed to obtain a lens with a given *front* vertex power (the preferred designation for near work lenses), and if important a modification must be made in the power ordered. See Chapter VI—Optics.

    4. In one piece or cemented high add bifocals one may specify upon which surface the segment is to be placed. Slightly more magnification results if the segment is placed on the front surface (Wild, 1968).

    5. In arriving at the final lens form, the practitioner must balance the factors of weight, cosmetics, and economics versus the patient's ability to benefit from any theoretical improvement due to superior optics.

D. Centering

    1. Because of increased aberrations, restricted fields, and induced prismatic effects, special attention must be given to securing the proper centering of low vision aids. Both the horizontal and vertical location of the centers should be designated.

    2. Where high power microscopic lenses are used, the center may have to be dropped in order to compensate for the normal tendency to hold near targets in an inferior position.

    3. Some practitioners use direct observation to measure the proper lens centration. After the patient is fitted with a frame, a piece of transparent tape is placed over the lens aperture. A mark is then placed on the tape in line with the apparent center of the cornea or pupil. This method does not account for errors where the visual axis does not pass through the center of either the cornea or pupil because of physiological or pathological fixation.

    4. Subjective methods of determining proper lens centration are usually much more reliable

MONOCULAR DECENTRATION FOR NEAR ADDS

Dist. PD	58 mm.	60 mm.	62 mm.	64 mm.	66 mm.	68 mm.	70 mm.	72 mm.
ADD + 4.00D.	2.6 mm.	2.7 mm.	2.8 mm.	2.9 mm.	3.0 mm.	3.1 mm.	3.2 mm.	3.3 mm.
+ 5.00D.	3.2	3.3	3.5	3.6	3.7	3.8	3.9	4.0
+ 6.00D.	3.8	3.8	4.1	4.2	4.3	4.5	4.6	4.7
+ 7.00D.	4.3	4.5	4.6	4.8	4.9	5.1	5.2	5.4
+ 8.00D.	4.8	5.0	5.2	5.3	5.5	5.7	5.9	6.0
+ 9.00D.	5.3	5.5	5.7	5.9	6.1	6.2	6.5	6.6
+10.00D.	5.8	6.0	6.2	6.4	6.6	6.8	7.0	7.2
+11.00D.	6.3	6.5	6.7	6.9	7.1	7.4	7.6	7.8
+12.00D.	6.7	6.9	7.2	7.4	7.6	7.9	8.1	8.3

Fig. XI-1.   Chart of monocular decentration for near adds. These figures only consider the decentration required for the near interpupillary distance. Any decentration to create base-in prism must be added to the above. Calculations assumed that the object is in the primary focal plane of the add and the center of rotation of the eye is 2.5cm. behind the spectacle plane.

than direct observation methods. One may devise an anaglyph system using polaroid or mutually exclusive transmission filters (Red-Green, Blue-Yellow, etc.) over the selected frame with an appropriately designed fixation target. Engelmann (1961) has designed such a system for proper near lens centering which is available from Designs for Vision. This can also be used for distance centering by adding the proper distance target.

5. Binocular centering

   a. Where binocular vision is to be attempted, precise decentration is required (see Figure XI-1). The decentration may not be equal in the two lenses.

   b. Ideal centration required to minimize aberration effects may have to be modified because base-in prism usually must be incorporated into the prescription to help compensate for the increased demands on convergence required by the very short working distances (see Figures VIII-4 and VIII-5).

E. Position of Various Elements

   1. Insert telescopes

   a. The position of the telescopic system in the carrier lens should be measured under the conditions of use considering posture, head position, eccentric fixation, task requirements, etc.

   b. The anaglyph system discussed above is probably the preferred method to obtain proper centering even for a monocular device.

c. For binocular vision to be possible, the tubes must be angled for the specific fixation distance as well as any unusual vertical level of fixation. These notations must be specified in order.

2. Bifocal microscopics

a. Bifocal segments should be set unusually high unless distance vision requirements are primary. Some authorities recommend positioning the segment as if it were a trifocal. Others have obtained excellent results positioning the segment line at the upper margin of the pupil with the eye in the primary position and illumination approximating the conditions of use. The stronger the add and the lower the optical center within the segment, the higher the segment must be set.

b. As in the case of telescopics, precise binocular decentration is required in those instances in which binocular vision is to be attempted. Figure XI-1 gives the decentrations required for various adds and interpupillary distances.

c. Where base-in prism is incorporated, the decentration should be adjusted to compensate for the reduced angle of fixation through the prism (see Figure XI-2).

The following formula can be used to calculate the decentration adjustment when base-in prism is incorporated:

$$Y = \frac{t\Delta}{100}$$

Y = change in centering required by prism (mm.)

t = distance from spectacle plane to center of rotation (positive; mm.)

Δ = prism (base-in : negative, base-out: positive; prism diopters)

Verification

General

Because of their complexity and unusual nature, many low vision aids require special verification techniques. One can no more assume infallibility and consistency for the low vision laboratory than one can for the regular ophthalmic or contact lens laboratory.

Frame

The following aspects should be inspected and verified:

A. Color

B. Size

C. Workmanship

D. Alignment

Lens System

A. Surface defects

Examine surfaces both by reflected and transmitted light.

B. Clarity and uniformity of media

Examine for liquid or stray cement between or on lenses.

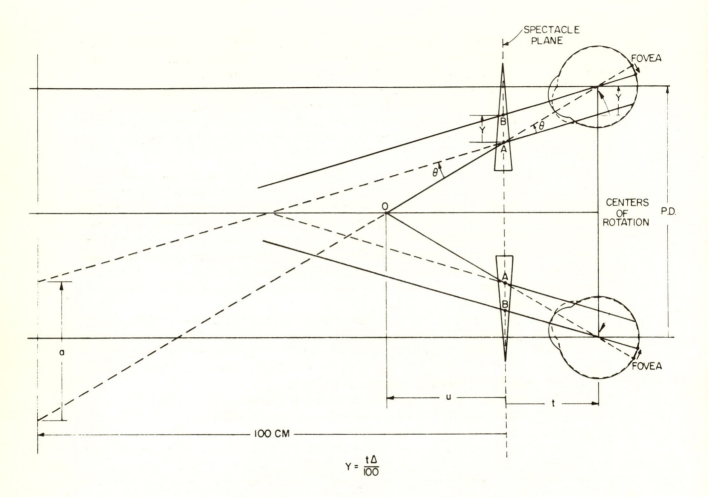

$$Y = \frac{t\Delta}{100}$$

Fig. XI-2.   *Diagram showing decentration correction required for bifocal segments with base-in prism. Light rays emanating from the object, O, are deflected by the prism through the angle θ, requiring that the eye turn outward. The new line of sight intersects the spectacle plane at a point θ, displaced distance Y from the intersection point A without prism.*

C. Stability of elements

Elements of multiple and single lens units should be checked for tightness and immobility in the carrier (if any) and frame.

D. Ametropia correction and magnification

1. Microscopic spectacles

a. When a single vision lens is ordered in diopters, the laboratory will customarily supply the power calculated in terms of *back* focal length and the lens received should be verified in that manner.

b. When a lens is ordered in magnification power (✕), the laboratory should supply a lens whose *front* focal power (in diopters) is four times the magnification power ordered and the lens received should be verified in that manner.

c. When a lens has been ordered as a distance correction with a near add, the distance correction is in terms of *back* focal length while the near add is in terms of *front* focal length. To verify these aspects separately, the procedure is as follows. Either neutralize the add ordered with trial lenses at the front surface then measure the *back* vertex power. This measures the ametropic correction. Or, measure the *front* vertex power while holding the lenses to neutralize the ametropia correction against the ocular surface of the system. This is a measure of the near add. To change this dioptric power to "effective" magnification divide by four.

d. Where the lens power to be measured is beyond the range of the focometer, the lens to be measured is placed in the instrument and the auxiliary concave lenses placed in contact with the exposed surface. A simple method of determining the power effect of the auxiliary concave lens *in this location* is to "read" the scale power after removing the microscopic while retaining the concave lens in its original position. The power effect of the auxiliary lens is subtracted algebraically from the scale reading when measuring the microscopic lens.

e. In those instances where a device will not fit into a focometer, hand neutralization or optical bench technique can be used.

2. Magnifiers, loupes, etc.

a. Because of the factors discussed in this chapter under Fitting and Ordering, *Lens Specifications* (B-5), the surest designation of these devices is in terms of front vertex dioptric power, lens diameter, lens material, lens form, carrier, and manufacturer and stock number, if known, e.g. +5.00 D., 3-⅞″ × 2″, glass, spherical, self-illuminated, hand held magnifier, black plastic handle, XYZ Optical Company #106.

b. In verifying magnifiers all the above factors should be checked.

3. Telescopes

a. Ametropia correction

If the prescription is removable it is easily evaluated in a focometer, remembering to verify that the telescope is afocal after the ametropia correction has been removed.

For non-removable prescriptions, one may place the entire telescope in the focometer with the ocular lens against the focometer stop. If a near add is also incorporated one must place a concave spherical lens of appropriate dioptric power for the working space (e.g. for 40 centimeters, –2.50 D.) against the objective lens while verifying the ametropia correction.

b. Near additions

Removable "caps" are readily verified by measuring their *front* vertex power in a focometer. Non-removable additions may be verified by placing the entire device in the focometer with the objective surface against the focometer stop, if there is no ametropic correction included. When both ametropic correction and near addition co-exist, it is simplest to proceed as in 3a above, since the two spherical elements are interdependent and it is not possible to verify one without assuming the other unless the device is dismantled.

c. Magnification

Before verifying the angular magnification of a telescope, any ametropic correction must be neutralized by lenses placed against the ocular.

The simplest method of verifying the magnification of an unknown telescope is to match its magnification to that of a known telescope, if one is available.

There are two other methods which offer greater freedom.

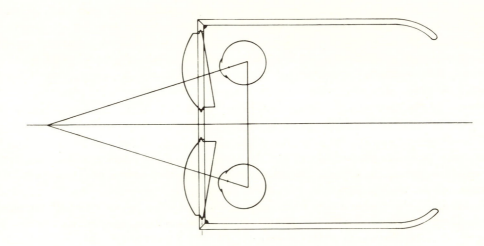

Fig. XI-3.   *Diagram showing angling of microscopic lenses for binocular use. This angling is necessary to allow the line of sight to pass perpendicularly through the principle planes of the lens, thus preventing the induction of unwanted cylindrical power.*

The first is: the measured diameter of the objective can be compared to the measured diameter of the objective's image as viewed through the ocular. Thus:

$$M = \frac{\text{Diameter of Objective}}{\text{Diameter of Eye Ring (image of objective by ocular)}}$$

The second method is: the linear size of a calibrated target, such as a meter stick, may be compared to the apparent linear size as seen through the telescope.

Illumination Elements
When present, illumination elements should be checked for proper functioning.

Dispensing and Adjusting

General
Sufficient time must be allowed for dispensing, not only to insure the proper fitting of a low vision device, but also to allow for further counseling in its care and use. The practitioner may again review when and how to use the aid, its limitations, and last but not least, care and cleaning of the device.

Instructions and demonstrations should include putting on and removing the device as well as the use of any removable or movable parts (e.g. illumination controls). Multiple lens units must not be immersed in or sprayed with liquids lest the air spaces may be infiltrated resulting in liquid stains even after drying.

Adjusting

A. General

With a good observer subjective methods are advantageous. As changes are made in the position of the aid, the patient's subjective responses are elicited and the frame parts are adjusted so that the frame will stay in that position which affords the best visual performance.

B. Telescopes

1. Insert systems should be adjusted for the height and angle affording the greatest ease of use.

2. Where binocular vision is expected, one may utilize a spot of light and red-green glasses to align the elements for easy fusion.

3. Pantascopic angle can be adjusted by having the patient observe bowing of a straight-edge seen through the telescopes. The angle is adjusted until the edge appears straight.

C. Microscopes

1. With the high powers usually involved, proper lens positioning is extremely important. Ideally the line of fixation should pass perpendicularly through the lens plane at the optical center.

With binocular vision, this may involve angling the lenses to make the temporal vertex distance greater than the nasal (see Figure XI-3).

2. Bifocal microscopes should be adjusted so that the segment is high. See the section in this chapter on Fitting and Ordering Lens Specifications (E-2).

D. Comfort

Once the proper position of the aid has been attained, the practitioner should carefully inspect all bearing areas (nose and ears) to insure even distribution of weight and pressure. Ancillary frame devices may be used where necessary to assure comfort and stability

Chapter 12

Contact Lenses

General

This chapter will only discuss the use of contact lenses in low vision care. Techniques of fitting the lenses, including the specialized ones, are adequately covered in texts on contact lenses and will not be repeated here.

Although the role of contact lenses as low vision aids is limited, it can be a very significant one. In keratoconus, the vision improvement with contact lenses may be so great that the patient is not considered to be in the low vision category any longer. There are a small number of other patients for whom contact lenses produce much better visual acuity than any spectacles.

The use of a contact lens as the eyepiece of a Galilean telescope created a great deal of interest and experimentation in the late 1950's and early 1960's, but the number of successful cases has been disappointing. It is possible that some new technology or design may revive this idea in the future.

Conventional Lenses

The conventional contact lens has applicability in a number of conditions.

Keratoconus

Hard contact lenses, by providing a regular refractive surface to replace the irregular cornea as the anterior refracting element of the eye, produce great improvements in visual acuity. Furthermore, their use may prevent further progression of the cone.

Irregular Astigmatism and Corneal Scarring

Hard contact lenses function here in the same manner as they do in keratoconus to provide a regular refractive surface which may greatly improve visual acuity. When astigmatism is limited in amount, soft contact lenses may serve as well or even provide better acuity than hard lenses. Where a damaged cornea is being fitted, special care must be exercised to be certain that it will

145

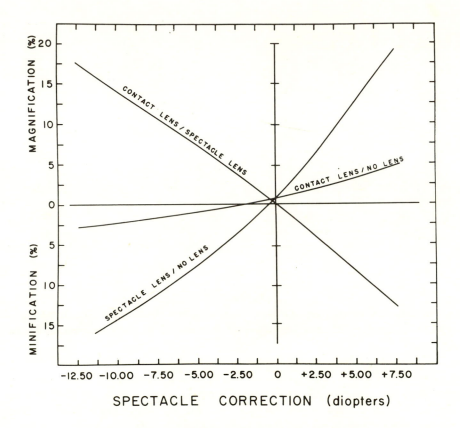

Fig. XII-1.   *Magnification of contact lenses and spectacle lenses. Effectivity has been allowed for so that all points on a vertical line refer to the same ametropia. (After Westheimer, 1962; reproduced by permission of The Journal of the American Optometric Association.)*

tolerate a contact lens. This is especially true for those instances where the cornea may be desensitized and corneal insult may not give rise to warning symptoms.

High Myopia
The high myope is classically recognized as a good candidate for contact lenses.

A. Magnification

Spectacle lenses produce minification (compared to unaided vision) in myopia. The amount of this minification is greatly reduced by contact lenses. Therefore, relative to a spectacle correction for myopia, the contact lens produces a magnified image on the retina (see Figure XII-1). Mandell (1965) calculates that a contact lens correction for a 15.00 D. myope would produce a 19.5% larger image on the retina than a spectacle correction at a vertex distance of 13 mm.

B. Aberrations

A stable, well centered contact lens can enhance vision by elimination of peripheral distortions and prismatic effects encountered in strong spectacles.

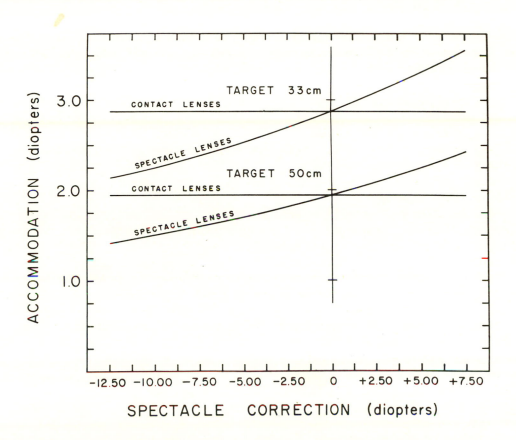

Fig. XII-2.   Accommodation required with contact lenses and spectacle lenses. Calculations assumed a spectacle plane 14 mm. in front of the cornea. (After Westheimer, 1962; reproduced by permission of The Journal Of The American Optometric Association.)

C. Near Vision

More accommodation is required to focus the eye-lens optical system for near distances when the myope is corrected with contact lenses than when he uses spectacles (see Figure XII-2). Moreover, many high myopes take advantage of their "built-in magnifiers" to read at very close distances by removing their spectacles.

The removal and replacement of spectacles is much more readily accomplished than is the case with contact lenses. Consequently, some of the advantages gained by the myope for his distance vision may be lost again for his near vision when he uses contact lenses.

Some high myopes with low vision remove their contacts for prolonged periods of close work while others use microscopic spectacles to read with their contact lenses in place.

D. Field

The minification of spectacles relative to contact lenses means that a larger area of the object field is represented on the same area of retina. Since the peripheral areas may be seriously distorted with spectacle correction or limited by a frame or a lenticular lens, the contact lens may not produce a noticeable change in the size of the object field for the patient whose field is large in extent. However, where the field is drastically restricted, any optically induced reduction in the object field may be detrimental.

E. Cosmetics

The cosmetic and psychological advantages of contact lenses for the high myope may be the most important factor of all for many patients. Since high myopia usually starts early in life, and produces frequent changes in vision and lenses, the patient with this condition has frequently been emotionally traumatized by his affliction. The symbolic significance of being able to see without glasses may be extremely important to him.

Aphakia and High Hyperopia

The advantages of contact lenses for aphakia are well known. In monocular aphakia they may permit single binocular vision which could not be attained with spectacles. For the partially-sighted patient the pros and cons need to be weighed.

A. Magnification

The correction of aphakia with spectacles results in approximately 28% magnification. This is reduced to approximately 12% by the use of contact lenses. In the reduction of aniseikonia, the lesser magnification of the contact lens is an advantage. However, for the low vision patient, who may be essentially monocular or binocularly aphakic, the increased magnification of spectacles provides the greater advantage.

An inspection of Figure XII-1 shows that contact lenses produce minification relative to spectacles for correcting hyperopes. The amount of minification is directly proportional to the power of the spectacle correction when a contact lens is substituted for a spectacle lens.

B. Aberrations

For aphakes and hyperopes requiring strong corrections, a well centered contact lens can markedly reduce peripheral distortions. The ring scotoma caused by the base-in prism effect of convex spectacle lenses is eliminated, removing the "Jack-in-the-Box" phenomena where objects appear and disappear in the periphery as the eye moves behind a strong convex lens (see Figure VI-9).

C. Near vision

The hyperope will find his accommodation more effective through contact lenses (see Figure XII-2), than spectacles and hence will require a weaker lens for focusing his eye-lens system for the same distance when using contact lenses. In the case of a low vision hyperope this gain may be negated by the minification of the contact lens which necessitates a closer viewing distance to provide increased magnification.

D. Field

The object field of view of the aphakic eye corrected with spectacles is reduced approximately 28% by the magnification (relative to a non-aphakic eye). By reducing this magnification, the contact lens enlarges the extent of the object field relative to the field through a spectacle correction. Relative to the non-aphakic eye, the object field is still reduced by approximately 12% even with contact lenses.

In hyperopia this enlargement of the extent of the object field by contact lenses is also present, the amount increasing with the amount of the hyperopic correction.

E. Cosmetics

The cosmetic and psychological advantages of contact lenses are as great for the congenital cataract patient or very high hyperope, who has worn lenses from early childhood, as for the high myope. For the person becoming an aphake in his adult years, the psychological factors have to be evaluated on an individual basis.

High Astigmia

For high astigmia that is regular, and not related to keratoconus, the considerations are the same as for high myopia and high hyperopia. In hyperopic astigmia there will be meridional minification (compared to spectacle lenses) with contact lenses. In myopic astigmia there will be meridional magnification (compared to spectacle lenses) with contact lenses. Meridional aniseikonia is usually reduced by contact lenses and can result in greatly improving fusion.

Nystagmus

Abrams (1955), Grosvenor (1963), and Ludlam (1960) report on cases of nystagmus being reduced and visual acuity being increased by use of contact lenses. Mandell (1965) states that where nystagmus has a visual causation and contact lenses effectively correct the visual defect, the nystagmus may be reduced.

Soft Lenses

Therapeutic

In the presence of some active corneal diseases (e.g. bullous keratopathy) the use of soft contact lenses is the therapy of choice. In addition to the therapeutic advantages, the lens often provides an improved refracting surface with enhanced visual performance. In some instances of corneal dystrophy, soft lenses may provide better acuity than either hard contact lenses or spectacles.

Occasional Wear

A further advantage of a soft lens is realized by the patient who uses contact lenses occasionally. For the irregular wearer, a soft lens causes less adaptation problems than a hard lens.

Astigmatism

Astigmatism is essentially not corrected by soft lenses. If other factors dictate the use of soft lenses, it may be necessary to correct astigmatism by spectacles worn over the contact lenses.

Telescopics

The Contact Lens Telescope

The idea of using a contact lens as the eyepiece of a Galilean telescope has been reported in the literature as early as 1939 (Bettman and McNair, 1939). Ludlam (1960) published a report of cases and data on optical systems' characteristics. He used minimum clearance scleral lenses with high minus powers as the eyepiece and strong convex spectacles as the objectives.

A. Optical specifications (Ludlam, 1960)

Using a –40.00 D. contact lens, a +26.30 D. spectacle lens at a vertex distance of 13 mm. will produce 1.52× magnification and a total field, with a 44 mm. eyesize in the spectacle, of 79 degrees. Increasing the vertex distance to 23 mm. would reduce the objective to +21.10 D., increase magnification to 1.91× and reduce the field to 43 degrees.

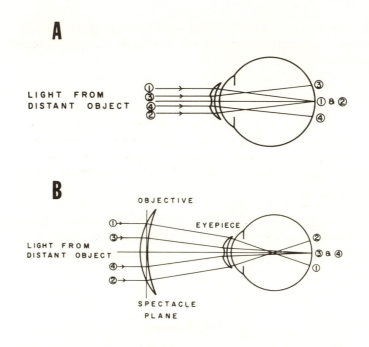

Fig. XII-3. *Diagram of bivisual contact lens telescope designed by Voss.*

A. Use as a normal contact lens for correction of ametropia. Rays 1 and 2 form a sharp image on the retina, while rays 3 and 4 are grossly out of focus on the retina.

B. Use of a contact lens as the eyepiece of a telescopic system. Rays 3 and 4 form a sharp, magnified image on the retina, while rays 1 and 2 are grossly out of focus on the retina.

(After Mandell, 1965; reproduced by permission of Charles C. Thomas, Publisher.)

A –30.00 D. contact lens, a +21.80 D. spectacle lens and a vertex distance of 13 mm. gives a magnification of 1.35× and a field of 87 degrees.

B. Advantages

1. There is a larger field of view compared to telescopic spectacles. Because of aberrations, the useful field is less than the total field. Mandell (1965) points out that using a 25 mm. lenticular lens as the objective only reduces the useful field a small amount, still leaving it larger than a telescopic spectacle.

2. The cosmetic appearance is a great improvement over a full field telescopic spectacle.

C. Disadvantages

1. The practical range of magnifications is limited.

2. Movement of the contact lens causes an apparent movement of the visual field.

3. Most of the disadvantages of full field telescopics, rapid movement of the visual field with head movements, telescopic parallax, etc. are also present with contact lens telescopes.

4. The strongly convex spectacle lenses are not cosmetically attractive and may be uncomfortable.

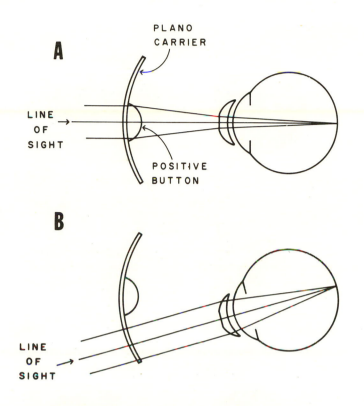

Fig. XII-4. *Diagram of Filderman's Telecon system.*
A. Use of a contact lens as the eyepiece of a telescopic system with a convex button on a spectacle lens as the objective.
B. Use as a normal contact lens for correction of ametropia by directing the line of sight away from the convex button and through the plano carrier portion of the spectacle lens.
(After Mandell, 1965; reproduced by permission of Charles C. Thomas, Publisher.)

5. The spectacles must be kept in very precise adjustment.

6. Accommodation is relatively ineffective so clip-ons or separate reading lenses are generally required for near vision.

7. When a non-magnified view is desired, the contact lens must be removed.

The Bivisual Contact Lens Telescope

Mandell (1965) reports on a bivisual system designed by Voss in 1958. This modification of the contact lens telescope was designed for use as a normal contact lens (by removing the spectacles) or as a telescope with the spectacles. This was accomplished by having a strong concave lens segment in the center of a contact lens which corrected the patient's ametropia (see Figure XII-3). The primary disadvantage of any bivisual system is that because of its design the performance of both optical systems is impaired. The light rays outside the concave segment will be lost to the eye when the telescope is used and those striking the concave segment lost when the non-telescopic

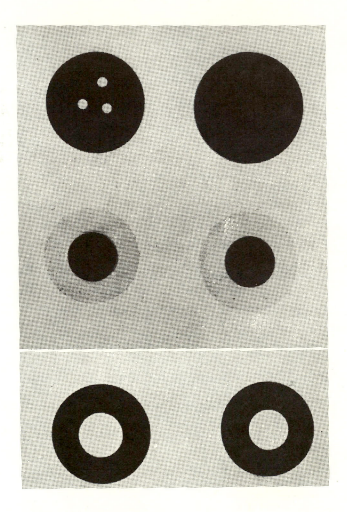

Fig. XII-5.   Controlled pupil contact lenses.
  Top, left : multi-pinhole contact lens.
  Top, right : totally opaque occluder contact lens.
  Middle : cosmetic contact lens with clear periphery and opaque pupil.
  Bottom : controlled pupil contact lenses with opaque periphery and transparent central optical zone.
  (After Rosenbloom, 1969; reproduced by permission of The Journal of the American Optometric Association).

system is used. Furthermore, the out of focus rays will produce a veiling effect which further reduces contrast of the retinal image. Most low vision patients require increased contrast and do very poorly with decreased contrast.

The Telecon System
Filderman (1959) improved on the bivisual system by using a flat area (for the ocular) on the front

of the contact lens. He recommended a diameter of 2.5 mm. The objective lens was incorporated in a segment of 10 mm. diameter centrally on the back of a plano spectacle lens (see Figure XII-4A).

While this reduces the telescopic field of view, it also permits an unmagnified field by turning eye or head and looking around the convex button (see Figure XII-4B).

Bifocals can be provided by using two convex buttons.

Telescopic in a Contact Lens
Feinbloom (1960) developed a telescope completely contained in a contact lens. It protruded further than a fluid scleral lens and was extremely difficult to wear and to fit.

Minifying Telescopic
The use of a reverse Galilean telescope to enlarge the object field for those patients having constricted fields but good visual acuity is discussed in Chapter X—Helping the Patient with a Visual Field Limitation. This type of device can be designed with the ocular a convex contact lens and the objective, a concave spectacle lens. The limitations discussed in Chapter X, as well as those discussed above for contact lens-spectacle telescopic systems apply.

Artificial Pupils
The Pupilens was described by Mazow (1958). Rosenbloom (1969) has reported on its use as a low vision aid (see Figure XII-5).

Uses
A. Overly large pupil as in aniridia, complete permanent mydriasis, and coloboma of the iris
B. Distorted pupil
C. Scarred cornea
D. Diffuse corneal opacities
E. Multiple disseminated opacities of the media
F. Subluxation of the lens
G. To improve cosmesis of an unsightly eye

Fitting
The fitting procedure is outlined in Rosenbloom's (1969) article. He points out that: "The successful prescribing of controlled pupil contact lenses demands intelligent selection of patients, exacting visual analysis, and painstaking skill in fitting the contact lens."

Microscopics
The use of a strong convex contact lens as a microscopic system for near vision has been discussed by Bier (1970), Mandell (1965) and others. A single vision lens has to be removed whenever distance vision is required. Bifocal contact lenses present many problems. For the same power and magnification, microscopic contact lenses foreshorten the already short working distance of microscopic spectacles because of the loss of the vertex distance.

Chapter 13

Training

Introduction

The importance of proper training in the use of low vision aids cannot be overemphasized for *successful* vision rehabilitation. Many low vision devices that are unused, are rejected because of inadequate training.

One of the cardinal rules of successful low vision care is that *a patient must never be allowed to take a low vision device home until he can demonstrate that he is proficient in its use*. This rule applies even in the case of the most simple devices such as typoscopes or hand held magnifiers.

Even those applications of aids and procedures which seem fundamental and natural to the practitioner are, in fact, in many cases highly technical and complex to the patient. New sensory-motor coordination patterns of eye, head, hand, and body movements must be developed.

Many low vision patients, having experienced repeated failures, develop an attitude of expecting failure. They easily become frustrated and discouraged and will quickly accept failure rather than trying to work out the problem, regardless of how simple the solution may be. To send such a patient home with instructions to "try the aid and see if you can use it" is practically insuring rejection.

General Considerations

Working Distance
Patients are not accustomed to working at the distances imposed by most low vision aids. Patients must be trained in positioning and maintaining material at the proper distance for best vision.

Field of View
Most aids result in drastic reduction of the useable visual field, consequently, there are problems of mobility, orientation, scanning, and manipulation to be overcome.

Illumination

Because the illumination requirements of the partially-sighted may be so radically different from the generally held concept of optimum lighting, retraining is essential. To overcome these deep-seated attitudes and habits, the patient must be drilled in specific methods of obtaining the required illumination and controlling the lighting environment.

Aid Manipulation

The unusual characteristics of some aids combined with inability of some patients to read the accompanying instructions or to see the details of the aid itself, necessitates practice in handling the device. Often, non-visual manipulation must be planned and trained.

Physiological and Pathological Optics

Field Restriction

A very restricted central field, such as in glaucoma or retinitis pigmentosa, requires more head movements and less eye movements. Training time should emphasize this skill.

Central Scotomas

Loss of central vision, such as in macular degeneration and central chorioretinitis, will require increased scanning eye movements, and training should emphasize this skill. Loss of foveal vision may necessitate teaching eccentric viewing.

General Guidelines

Instructions

In order to afford the best chance of success, it is important that patients be given *complete* and *specific* instructions and be required to demonstrate understanding and proficiency in carrying out these instructions before being allowed to take any device for unsupervised use.

Structured Routine

A. Training procedures should follow a regular routine.

B. Training is most efficiently accomplished in daily sessions when possible, although alternate days can be used. The interval between sessions should be short so there will be a carry-over from one session to the next.

C. Duration of individual training sessions should be such as to avoid fatigue. One may begin with a quarter to a half hour per day.

D. When progress warrants, training may be continued at home. A third party (parent, spouse, friend, teacher, etc.) can be of great assistance if he understands the correct utilization of the aid. Caution should be exercised in choosing the out of office helper lest an adverse interpersonal relationship interfere with the training.

   1. The total training time may be increased slightly each day.

   2. Training is best divided into several short periods during the day rather than one long one.

   3. The patient, when fully proficient, may use the aid as long as he wishes as long as stress or fatigue do not develop.

E. Patients should be guided in the correct procedures, but most important, they must be given encouragement and *immediate* praise on their performance and progress even though at times the progress is minimal. Errors may be ignored and only correct performance praised or if an error persists, the preferred technique should be restated and practiced.

F. Periodic evaluations of the procedures and effects of training should be scheduled at regular intervals.

G. Training should follow the usual sequence for teaching motor skills:

1. *Motivation*

The patient not only must be motivated to develop a certain visual capability, but must understand the purpose of the specific skill he is learning and how it relates to the desired capability.

2. *Explanation*

3. *Demonstration*

4. *Practice*

5. *Transfer*

Clinically trained skills only have value when transferred to the patient's "real" life situation. Because a patient has learned to create the proper illumination in the office setting does not assure that he will understand how to create it in other settings. Additionally, he may have to acquire a new lamp and overcome his deeply ingrained previous habits. Consequently, training must include practice in the "real" setting.

Design of Exercises

A. At the beginning, the environment and difficulty of the task should be adjusted to make the goal easily attainable. Thus successful performance, as well as praise, becomes reinforcement of the desired behavior.

B. Gradually, the environment is made more normal and the task more difficult.

C. For example, training in reading

1. Begins with:

low magnification, large print, good contrast, widely spaced letters, short words, optimum illumination, and a typoscope.

2. Gradually introduces:

higher magnification, smaller print, poorer contrast, closer spacing, longer words, less controlled illumination, and increased manipulation.

Suitability of Materials

A. The material used for training should bear close relationship to the task goal of the patient.

1. If the task goal is sewing, training is carried on using sewing materials, not reading cards.

2. The *final* training materials should closely duplicate those to be used in the patient's everyday life. Thus, the task of threading a needle eventually must be trained using the needle eye and thread size of the "real life" situation.

B. Since most patients receive some training in reading, special attention must be paid to reading materials. The following must be considered:

1. Vocabulary

2. Reading level

3. Interest in subject matter

4. Ability to relate to subject matter

5. Ability to understand subject matter

36 Point

TO BE READ AT ___ INCHES FROM YOUR EYES

30 Point

Vision does not take place in the eyes. Vision takes place in the brain. The eyes are tools for the brain.

Display Advertising and Headlines

24 Point

They are like a factory. They convert one substance into another. They convert light into nervous energy which is carried by the optic nerves to be interpreted in the brain.

Display Advertising and Headlines

18 Point

There are changes in your eyes which interfere with this normal change over from the light image to an image of nerve impulses. That is why optical images which would be formed by glasses never get to your brain as well formed nervous impulse images.

Newspaper Headlines
Edward Goodlaw 1967

14 Point

Glasses as ordinarily fitted did not make you see adequately.
Your medical doctors have done all they could to cure the tissue defects in your eyes, but such help is obviously not possible.

Nevertheless, reading can be brought into your reach by supplying strong light to create a strong optical picture on the back of your eye and magnifying it enough.

Children's Book.

12 Point

Magnification will bridge the gap created by the defects in your eyes.
Magnification is spreading the image from working tissue to other healthy working tissue. Thus, the letters which are too small for you to read will be magnified to the size of the bigger

newspaper headline letters which you can read. However, the mechanics of a magnified world instead of the visual world to which you have been accustomed is going to present a learning challenge to you.

Books

10 Point

You have to learn to use this optical device if you are to reap its benefits. In optics, increased magnification means a reduced field of view and closer focus. You will not be able to see as far to the side as you did before. You will have to learn to put together the letters into meaningful words as they appear to you in a smaller space and fewer letters at a time.

The magnification to increase the letter size will also magnify any movement of your head. If you attempt to read by turning your head as you read across the page, the letters will seem to fly past your eyes. Hold your head still and move the page slowly from right to left as you read it from left to right.

Newspaper

8 Point

Practice this over and over until you master this skill. Because this magnifying device requires you to hold reading material closer to your eyes, adapt yourself to this reading position. Don't fight it by even thinking your reading should be done at any other position. Slowly bring the reading material closer to your eyes until it appears clear and keep it at this position. Don't let fatigue make you drop your arms and move the page farther. The print will begin to blur as soon as you change this distance.

Brace yourself by resting your elbows against your sides so that you can hold your reading material to this exact distance from your eyes, with steadiness. If you are trying to read a newspaper or large magazine, fold it so you can easily hold it to this distance from your eyes. Practice, practice, practice, until it is your habit to bring what you are reading to this proper distance from your eyes for clearest vision. When this has become "natural" for you, you will read with ease.

Stock Reports & Phone Directory

6 Point

Don't forget the good strong light. The light should come from behind you and so positioned to illuminate the print well even though the page is close to your eyes.

Also turn the other lights on in the room. The room should be well lit, and the page you are reading about three or four times brighter than the light in the room.

Footnotes
Edward Goodlaw 1967

Practice over and over. You are learning to read again.

Fig. XIII-1. Goodlaw low vision training chart. The chart includes the following point type sizes: 36, 30, 24, 18, 14, 12, 10, 8 and 6. (Reproduced by permission of Edward Goodlaw.)

6. Impact of "messages" (see Chapter VII—The Low Vision Examination, Examination Procedures, *Subjective Testing* (A-2).

7. Age suitability

The most readily available reading material having large print, good spacing, good contrast, etc. is usually designed for beginning readers in primary grades. When this material is presented to an adult or older child, he may feel that he is being treated as a "six year old".

Goodlaw (1968) has devised some very helpful material for reading training for adults, which takes into account all of the above seven points as well as print size, spacing, contrast, size of words, etc. (see Figure XIII-1).

Specific Training

Telescopes

A. General

    1. Explain and demonstrate the problems and solutions to:

        a. Attaining the maximum improvement in visual discrimination

        b. Limitations of the field of view

            i. Teach the patient to use fewer eye movements substituting head movements or movement of the material viewed (as in reading).

            ii. Teach the patient how to locate the object of regard.

        c. Telescopic parallax

The patient must be taught to bring the object to be manipulated within his field of view before judging its distance from other objects within the field, e.g. to pick up an object from a table, the patient must have both his hands and the object within the telescopic field before attempting to make contact.

    2. Environment

The training material and environment should simulate the situation for which the telescope has been prescribed.

    3. Devices

In some cases it is best that early training be accomplished using the testing devices themselves. This eliminates pressure from the patient to take the device home before proficiency warrants it. Also, should training indicate an improvement over the intended prescription, this can be accomplished before the finished aid is ordered.

    4. Sequence

        a. The head and object are stationary.

        b. The head is stationary and the object moves.

        c. Both the head and the object move.

B. Partial field (insert) telescopes

Teach the patient when and how to use the telescopic and non-telescopic sections, e.g., using the carrier lens for walking and the insert telescope for reading a sign.

C. Hand or stand held telescopes

    1. The patient must learn to hold the telescope as close to the eye as possible.

    2. Proper alignment must be developed including lateral and vertical positioning as well as tilt angle.

3. Focusing procedures must be learned.
    a. changing ocular-objective distance
    b. adding auxiliary lenses to objective
D. Near vision
    1. Focusing for near (where necessary) must be learned as in C-3 above.
    2. Train the patient to achieve and maintain the proper working distance.

Microscopic Spectacles and Headborne Loupes

A. Working distance

Since strong convex lenses permit a small depth of focus with or without accommodation, working distance is extremely critical and the patient must learn to control this distance exactly. Korb (1972) recommends that the presbyopic patient begin with the material at his nose and slowly move it out until it comes into focus. The authors have found this technique very useful in overcoming patients' resistance to decreasing their habitual working distance. When the patient reports the print "fading away" the doctor or assistant should remind him to move it closer to bring it back into focus.

B. Positioning material

    1. The material should be angled so as to be parallel to the lens plane.

    2. Because of peripheral aberrations, vision will be better if the patient looks through the center of the lenses. Thus, he must be taught to hold the material higher than the usual reading position. He should also move the material or his head laterally so as to keep the material near the lateral center of the lens.

C. Localization (applies also to telescopes for near)

    1. The limited field of view causes difficulties in locating material and in following a line of print once it has been located. Even more difficulty is encountered in switching from the end of the line to the beginning of the next.

    2. A typoscope, straight edge, or finger are helpful with these problems and should always be used in early training. Before the guide is discarded, a patient should learn the technique of quickly retracing (visually) from right to left the line just completed and when the first word is reached dropping his gaze to the next line.

D. Illumination

    1. Due to the short working distance illuminating reading material usually presents a physical problem.

    2. The patient must be coached in the proper use of goose-neck and high intensity lamps.

Hand or Stand Held Magnifiers

A. Location of magnifier

The same retinal image size can be maintained with any eye to lens distance, however decreasing this distance decreases the effects of aberrations and markedly increases the field of view. The patient should be taught how he may increase his working distance if he maintains the object in the focal plane of the lens or how he can improve the clarity and field size by decreasing the eye to lens distance. One should demonstrate the practical applications of this flexibility.

B. Location of material

The patient should be shown the outer (primary focal plane) and inner limits of object to lens distance and that for any given eye to lens distance, the largest retinal image is obtained when the object approaches the outer limit.

C. Angle

The material and lens must be in parallel planes, even with *fixed* stand magnifiers, and the patients often require training in this skill and in developing the proper sighting angle.

D. Movement

Frequently patients require practice in lateral and vertical manipulation of the magnifier to bring material into view in the proper sequence.

Illumination Controls

A. General

Although most illumination controls are relatively simple and easy to use, we cannot assume that patients, especially the elderly, will understand their function and proper use. Because they have not been properly indoctrinated in their importance, and consequently are not impressed with the benefits to be gained from an inexpensive piece of cardboard or plastic, many patients fail to use some of the simplest devices. Usually this training involves relatively little time, however it is still very important.

B. Lamps

Patients must be told specifically which lamp to use (and where to get it), which bulb to incorporate, where to place the lamp, and how to point it. Furthermore, they should practice until they demonstrate facility in proper utilization.

C. Visors, shields, slits, holes and typoscopes

The function of these devices must be understood by the patient. He also must demostrate that he can use and manipulate them properly.

Non-Optical Aids

Devices such as check stencils, self-threading needles, table easels, etc. require explanation and simple training just as has been indicated for illumination controls.

Chapter 14

Optical Aids

General

Seldom do two low vision practitioners use exactly the same aids and equipment. Success in patient care is not only determined by special techniques, but also to a considerable extent by the knowledge of the various parameters of the aids as well as their individual peculiarities.

This chapter is an attempt to describe some of the aids more commonly used in the United States. The list of aids discussed is by no means complete, and the omission of a particular aid from inclusion does not imply a lack of merit for that aid. The aids which are discussed are those with which the authors are more familiar.

The specifications for the aids discussed are those given by the individual manufacturer unless otherwise noted. As has been pointed out elsewhere in this book, because many aids are not primarily supplied through ophthalmic distributors, and because specifications are changed without notice, it is important that the low vision practitioner evaluate each aid as it is received for testing or prescribing so that he will be aware of the true characteristics of a specific aid.

Telescopes

Clip-on Telescopes

A. Aloe

The Albert Aloe Company produces two clip-on telescopic units (see Figure XIV-1). The "Distance Unit" is specified at 2.5× magnification while the "Reading Unit" is specified as producing 2.2× magnification. The distance unit is focusable and the reading unit is non-focusable and set for seven to nine inches.

With print at 7½ inches from the cornea, the authors viewed a field of 15° (as wide as the average news column).

B. Selsi

The Selsi Company imports and supplies a clip-on monocular which can also be obtained through several other distributors (see Figure XIV-2). The magnification specified is 2.5×. The telescope is focusable and also comes with an adapter to hold near addition lenses. The authors viewed a 10° field through the device set for distance.

The clip-on wire can be removed from the telescope, in which case it may be used as a hand-held device.

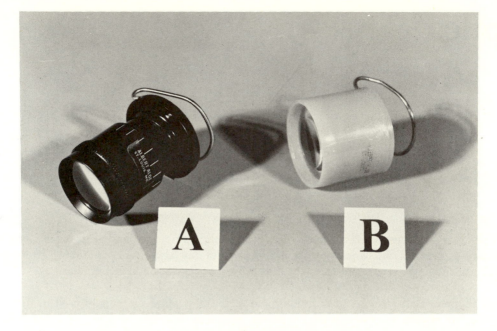

Fig. XIV-1.   *Aloe clip-on telescopes.*
   A.   Distance unit.
   B.   Reading unit.

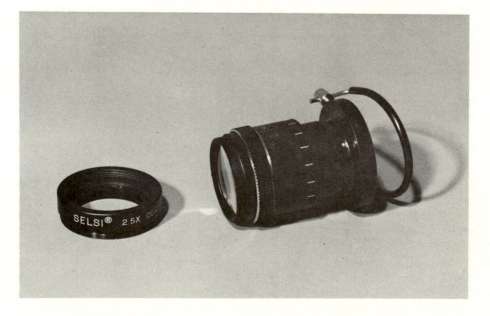

Fig. XIV-2.   *Selsi clip-on telescope with adapter for near addition lenses.*

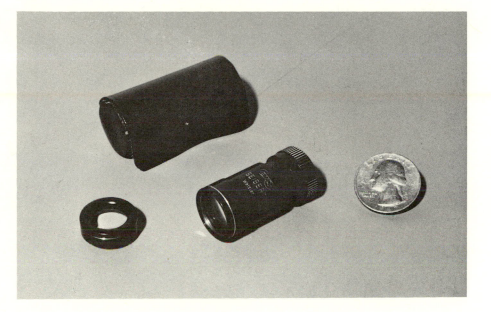

Fig. XIV-3.   *Emoskop with near lens adapter and carrying case. A twenty-five cent coin is shown for size comparison.*

Hand-Held Telescopes

To review all the available hand-held telescopes (binoculars and monoculars) in a book of this size is not possible. Thus, the following is a list only of those which the authors have found most useful. Many clip-on and head-borne telescopes can be readily separated from their clips or mountings and thus become hand-held. Those devices will not be reviewed in this section as they are discussed under their own sections of clip-on and head-borne telescopes.

A. Binoculars

Since most low vision patients have unequal visual function of the two eyes, and thus receive monocular aids, only single hand-held telescopes (monoculars) will be described in this chapter. In those cases where binocularity is possible and preferred and where the duration of their use is not restricted by their weight, binoculars may be prescribed. There are many such devices available from various manufacturers and importers such as Bausch & Lomb, Bushnell, Selsi, Zeiss, etc.

The specifications of the individual binoculars are readily available in the manufacturer's literature and most times are also imprinted on the binoculars themselves.

B. Monoculars

1. Emoskop

The Emoskop is a 2.5× monocular telescope available from Ocular Instruments Company (see Figure XIV-3). It is only 1¾ inches long and ¾ inch in diameter, hence easily carried in the hand. It is focusable (sliding action) and also has a near lens adapter of approximately +40.00 diopters, which should be removed to use the telescope as a low vision aid. The authors viewed the field to be 10° when set for distance. Included with it is a small leather carrying case.

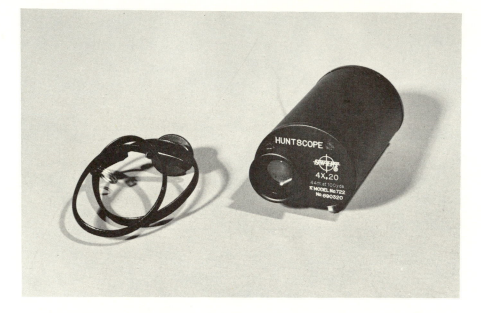

Fig. XIV-4.   Huntscope with carrying strap. The pocket clip attached to the underside of the telescope is not visible in the photograph.

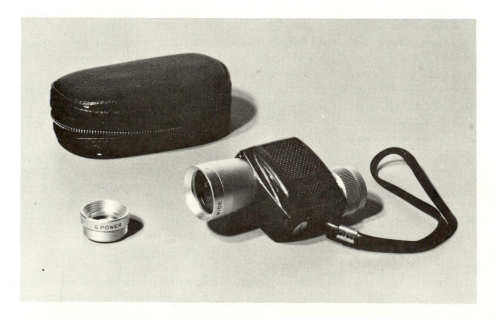

Fig. XIV-5.   Miniscope with 8X objective attached. The alternate 6X objective and carrying case are also shown.

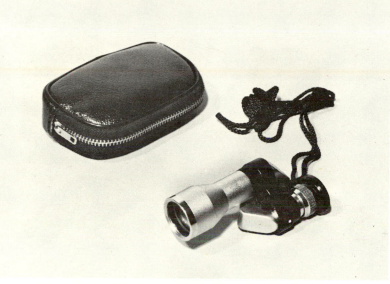

Fig. XIV-6.   Miniature monocular, 10X20mm. with carrying case.

2. Huntscope

The Huntscope, by Swift Instruments Incorporated, is specified as a 4×20 mm. monocular (see Figure XIV-4). It is 3½ inches long, has a fixed focus from 50 feet to infinity and is rated as having a 16.6° field.

3. Miniscope

The Miniscope by Selsi is a convertible 6×18 mm., 8×24 mm. prismatic monocular (see Figure XIV-5). The conversion is made by an exchange of objective systems which easily screw into the housing. Specifications detail that when it is a $6 \times$ system, it has an 11° field while when an $8 \times$, an 8.2° field. When $6 \times$, its overall length is 2⅞ inches, while when $8 \times$, it is 3½ inches. By adjusting the ocular lens system, it is focusable to as close a distance as 25 feet for $8 \times$ and 12 feet for $6 \times$. By unscrewing the objective system, these distances may be reduced to 8 feet and 3½ feet respectively. It has a wrist strap attached and is furnished with a carrying case. Similar devices are available from Bushnell and Colonial Optical.

4. Miniature monocular

Selsi has available both 6×15 mm. and 10×20 mm. miniature prismatic monoculars (see Figure XIV-6). The $6 \times$ is 2⅛ inches long and the $10 \times$ is 3¼ inches long. Both monoculars are focusable; the $6 \times$ as close as 17 feet and the $10 \times$ as close as 31 feet. As in the case of the Miniscope, the viewing distance can be considerably decreased by unscrewing the objective, the $10 \times$ decreasing to 12 feet. The $6 \times$ is rated as allowing a 14° field, while the $10 \times$ allows a 4° field. These monoculars are furnished with a neck string and a carrying case.

A similar 10×20 mm. monocular is available from Edmunds Scientific which can be focused as close as 15 feet normally and as close as 7½ feet by unscrewing the objective.

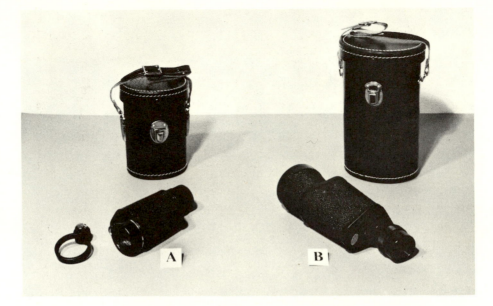

Fig. XIV-7.   *Prism monoculars with carrying cases.*
A.   6X30mm. with adapter for near addition lenses.
B.   7X50mm.

5. Prism monoculars

Prism monoculars in higher powers ($8\times$-$20\times$) generally can be used only for short periods unless a tripod is employed. Some patients are able to use lower powers to good advantage for longer periods when the weight of the aid is not too great. Selsi has the following available (see Figure XIV-7):

Size	Specified Field
6×30 mm.	7° 28′
8×30 mm.	7° 28′
7×35 mm.	6° 29′
7×50 mm.	7° 9′
10×50 mm.	5° 24′
12×50 mm.	5° 19′
16×50 mm.	4° 10′
20×50 mm.	3°
$7\times$ -$12\times$ 40 mm. zoom	Variable

These monoculars are designed for outdoor use and cannot be focused for close distances. All of these monoculars have adapters threaded for a tripod and are furnished with a stiff leather case. Similar as well as other types of monoculars are available from many other manufacturers and importers.

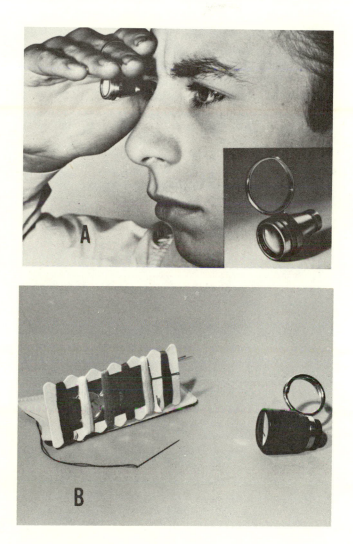

Fig. XIV-8.   Keeler ring telescopes.
   A.   2.3X15mm.
   B.   3.0X18mm. A needle and thread are shown for size comparison.

6. Ring telescopes

Keeler Optical Products supplies small telescopes mounted on finger rings. The telescopes are fixed focus for distance and small enough to be concealed in the palm of a cupped hand (see Figure XIV-8).

A small ring mounted telescope is also available from George Hellinger (see Figure XIV-9). This miniature telescope differs from the others in that it is focusable.

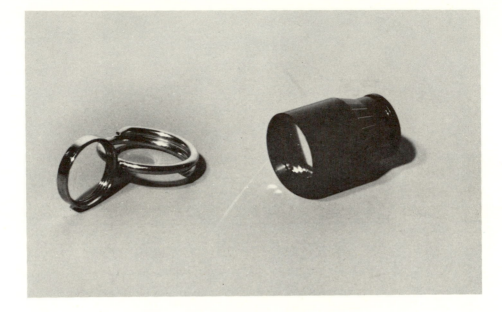

Fig. XIV-9.   Hellinger ring telescope, 3.0X18mm.

The authors found the three telescopes to have the following parameters:

Source	Magnification	Objective Diameter	Length	Focus	Clear Vision Range	Approximate Total Object Field
Keeler	2.3×	15 mm.	25 mm.	Fixed	Infinity to 11 feet	13.5°
Keeler	3.0×	18 mm.	31 mm.	Fixed	Infinity to 25 feet	12°
Hellinger	3.0×	18 mm.	24-27 mm.	Variable	Beyond infinity to 3 feet	11.5°

Headborne Telescopes

Selsi supplies headborne telescopes in two powers: 2.5× and 2.8× (see Figure XIV-10). Both Sport Spectacles offer individual focus and both pupillary and bridge adjustments. The 2.8× is equipped with soft rubber opaque side shields. Either device can be easily dismantled to provide two small monoculars. Both of these devices are supplied with a carrying case.

Various other binocular headborne telescopes for distance and near are available from other suppliers.

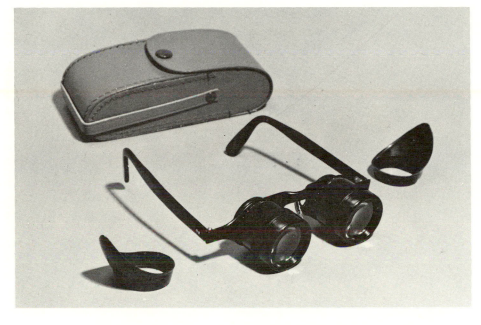

Fig. XIV-10.   *Selsi 2.8X sport spectacles with rubber side shields and carrying case.*

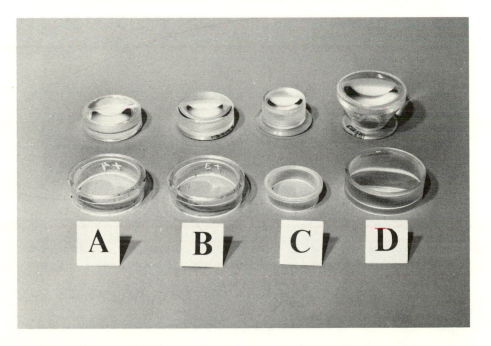

Fig. XIV-11.   *Feinbloom full field telescopes and representative near addition caps. The caps, front row, are sized to fit the objective of the telescope, rear row. A. 1.3X; B. 1.7X; C. 2.2X; D. 2.2X wide angle.*

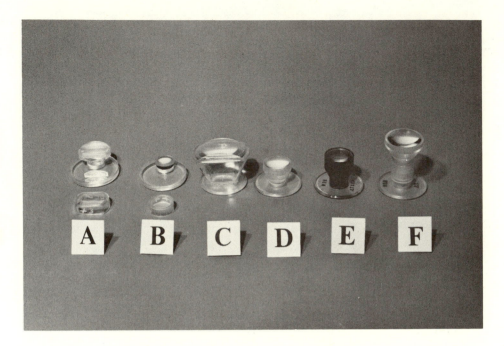

Fig. XIV-12.   Feinbloom insert type telescopes (bioptics).
A.   2.2X type I with near addition cap. The 1.7X is similar in appearance.
B.   2.2X type II with near addition cap.
C.   2.2X wide angle.
D.   3.0X
E.   4.0X
F.   6.0X

Prescription Telescopes

A. Designs for Vision

Designs for Vision produces and supplies telescopic spectacles designed by Dr. William Feinbloom. The telescopics, made of glass and plastic combination, are available in full diameter (see Figure XIV-11) or insert form (see Figure XIV-12). Bioptics feature a telescopic insert in a single vision lens, while trioptics feature an insert in a bifocal lens (see Figure XIV-13).

The magnification powers specified are: 1.3×, 1.7×, 2.2×, 3.0×, 4.0×, and 6.0×. Because of the loss of accommodation effect (see Chapter 6 - Optics), fixed focus telescopes of 3× and above have a negligible focal range even for distances usually considered essentially equal to infinity. Refractive error corrections may be incorporated into the telescopes as well as the carrier lenses. Near additions are available in the form of caps which slip over the front end of the telescope. Caps are available in full diameter or half lens form (telescopic bifocal).

The telescopic housings may be clear or black and lenses may be clear or tinted.

Also available is a binocular telescopic (Surgical Glasses) focused and angled for near distances (see Figure XIV-14). While the 2.5× binocular is normally set for 14 inches and the 3.5× and 4.5×

binoculars are normally set for 16 inches, these distances may be varied by special order to the manufacturers.

While looking through the telescopes, with fixed central fixation, and the telescopes held just grazing the eye lashes, the authors were able to view the following total fields:

Telescope Form	Specified Magnification		Approximate Total Object Field	
Full field	1.3×		41°	
	1.7×		37°	
	2.2×		21°	
	3.0×		11°	
	4.0×		8°	
	6.0×		4.5°	
Wide Angle Full Field	2.2×		23°	
	3.0×		12°	
Bioptic— Model I	2.2×		20.5°	horizontal
			14.5°	vertical
	3.0×		11°	round
	4.0×		8°	round
	6.0×		4.5°	round
Wide Angle Bioptic—Model I	2.2×		22°	horizontal
			11°	vertical
Bioptic—Model II	2.2×		18.5°	round
Surgical Binoculars	*Work Distance*		*Monocular*	
	2.5×	40cm.	6cm.	horizontal
			5cm.	vertical
	3.5×	35cm.	5cm.	round
	4.5×	40cm.	4cm.	round

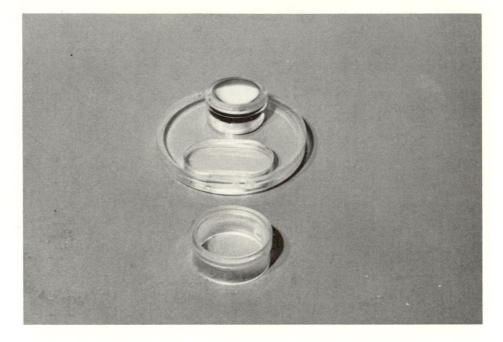

Fig. XIV-13.   Feinbloom insert type telescope mounted in a bifocal microscopic (trioptic). A near addition cap for the telescope is also shown. The telescope shown is 2.2X type II and the microscope is the "standard" type 13mm. by 23mm. The trioptic is also available with telescopes in powers 1.7X, 2.2X type I, 3.0X and 4.0X.

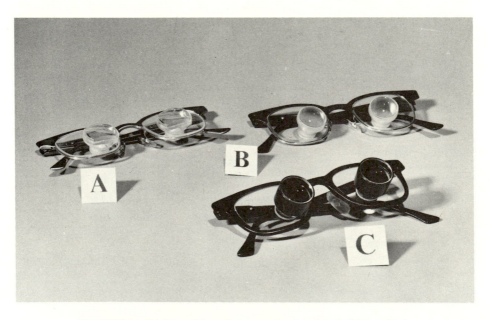

Fig. XIV-14.   Feinbloom binocular, near telescopes (surgical binoculars).
A.   2.5X; B. 3.5X; C. 4.5X.

B. Keeler Optical Products, Inc.

Keeler produces several models of telescopes, both for distance and near viewing. The telescopes are available mounted in three ways. The "standard" method involves the telescope being screwed into a holder which has been mounted to a standard frame by use of a locking ring. The "advanced" method involves the telescope being screwed into a sleeve which has been cemented to the front surface of a plastic lens containing the ametropic correction. The third method involves screwing the telescope into a bar which mounts in front of the frame. All three methods allow for interchanging telescopes when required.

The manufacturer lists the following telescopic devices and specifications:

Keeler L.V.A. Number	Method	Focus	Monocular or Binocular	Magnification	Form	Work Distance From Cornea (cm.)	Object Field	Comments
L.V.A.11	Std.	Dist.	Bino. or Mono.	2.5×	Insert			(see Figure XIV-15)
L.V.A.20	BAR	Dist.	Bino.	2×	BAR			(see Figure XIV-16)
L.V.A.20	Std.	Dist.	Mono.	2×	Insert			
L.V.A.21	BAR or ADV.	Near	Bino.	2× 3× 4× 5×	BAR or ADV.-insert	15.5 15.5 15.5 15.5	9.0 6.0 3.5 2.2	(See Figures XIV-17A and B).
L.V.A.21	Std. or ADV.	Near	Mono.	2× 3× 4× 5×	Insert	15.5 15.5 15.5 15.5	9.0 6.0 3.5 2.2	(See Figure XIV-18)
L.V.A.22	Std. or ADV.	Near	Bino.	1.6× 2×	Full Field	21.5 18.6	12.0 10.0	
L.V.A.22	Std. or ADV.	Near	Mono.	1.6× 2× 3× 4× 5× 6× 8×	Full Field	21.5 18.6 14.0 11.0 9.5 8.5 7.5	12.0 10.0 6.5 5.0 4.0 3.0 2.2	(See Figure XIV-19)
L.V.A.23	Std.	Dist. and Near	Dist. Mono Near: Bino. or Mono.	Dist: 2.5× Near: Bino 1.6×, 2× Mono. 1.6×, 2×, 3×, 4×, 5×, 6×	Dist-Insert Near-Full			(See Figure XIV-20) a bitelescopic unit with a distance telescope inserted into the upper section of a full field near telescope
L.V.A.26	Std.	Dist. Interm. Near	Mono.	Dist. 2× Interm. 2× Near 2.5×	Full Field			One ocular with three interchangeable objectives (see Figure XIV-21)
L.V.A.31	Std.	Dist. and Interm.	Bino. or Mono.	2×	Full Field			Focusable from 3 meters to infinity

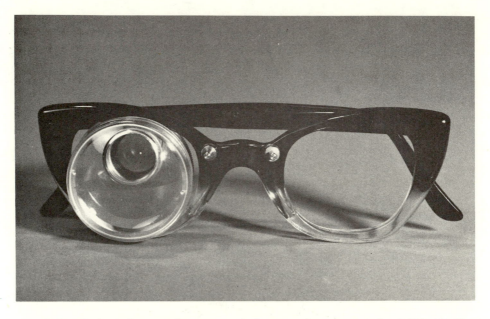

Fig. XIV-15. Keeler 2.5X monocular, insert type, distance, telescopic spectacles (L.V.A.-11). Photo courtesy of Keeler Optical Products, Inc.

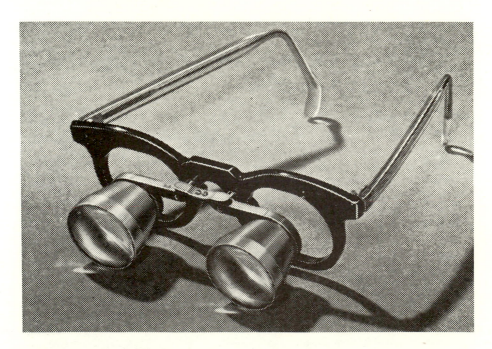

Fig. XIV-16. Keeler 2.0X binocular, bar type, distance, telescopic spectacles (L.V.A.-20). Photo courtesy of Keeler Optical Products, Inc.

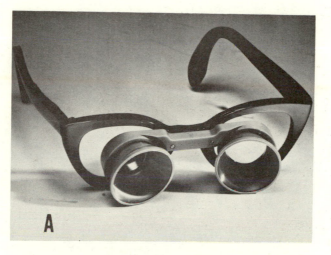

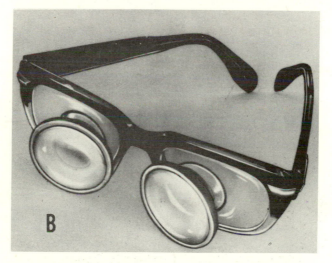

Fig. XIV-17.   Keeler binocular, near telescopic spectacles (L.V.A.-21).
   A.   Bar type.
   B.   Advanced method.
   Photo courtesy of Keeler Optical Products, Inc.

C. Zeiss

Carl Zeiss manufactures a full field telescopic spectacle system which produces a magnification of 1.8× with a 23 degree specified field of view. The ocular lenses are glass while the objective lenses and system housing are plastic (see Figure XIV-22). Ametropia corrections can be incorporated in the system and near addition caps are available in full diameter or half lens form (telescopic bifocal).

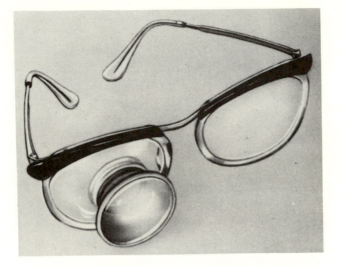

Fig. XIV-18.   Keeler monocular, near, insert type, telescopic spectacle, advanced method (L.V.A.-21). Photo courtesy of Keeler Optical Products, Inc.

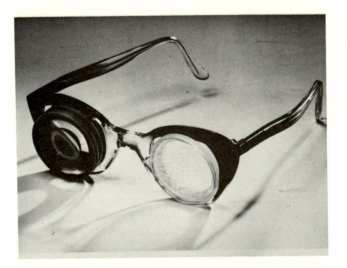

Fig. XIV-19.   Keeler monocular, near, full field, telescopic spectacle (L.V.A.-22). An occluder lens is shown in the left eyewire. Photo courtesy of Keeler Optical Products, Inc.

Zeiss also produces a reduced field telescopic which is specified at 2× magnification (see Figure XIV-23). The telescope is engaged with a ring according to the push-button principle. This ring is in turn cemented to the front of the carrier lens. This telescope is also available focused for either 20 or 33 cm. When set for 20 cm., the field is specified as 35 mm., while when set for 33 cm., the field is specified as 45 mm.

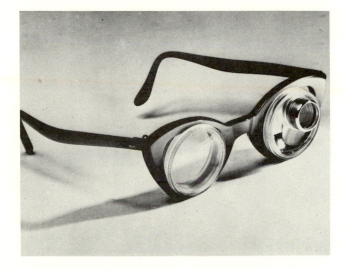

Fig. XIV-20.   Keeler binocular, near, full field, telescopic spectacle with a monocular, distance, insert type telescope (L.V.A.-23). Photo courtesy of Keeler Optical Products, Inc.

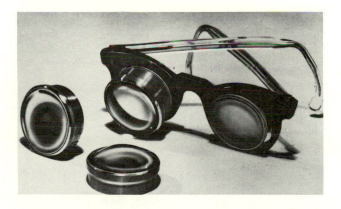

Fig. XIV-21.   Keeler monocular, full field, telescopic spectacle (L.V.A.-26). Objectives are interchangeable to focus for distance, intermediate, and near. Photo courtesy of Keeler Optical Products, Inc.

Microscopics

American Bifocal Company

American Bifocal Company supplies glass aspheric lenses for near work called Volk Conoid Lenses (see Figure XIV-24). The lenses are available in powers of +15D., +20D., +25D., +30D., +35D., +40D., +50D., +60D., +80D., and +100D. In all but the higher three powers, the lenses are available in finished or semi-finished form allowing the incorporation of cylindrical

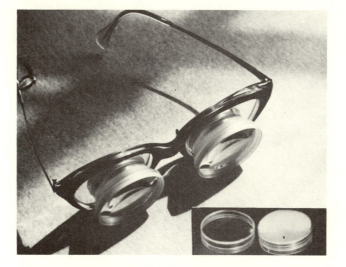

Fig. XIV-22.   *Zeiss full field 1.8× telescopic spectacles. Insert shows near addition cap and occluder cap. Photo courtesy of Carl Zeiss.*

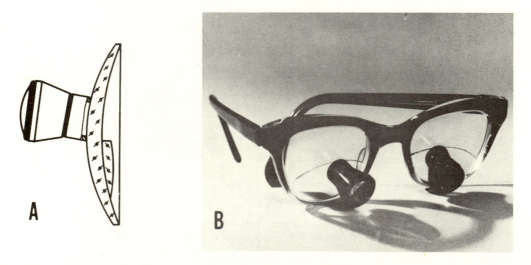

Fig. XIV-23.   *Zeiss reduced field 2X telescope.*
A.   Line drawing of telescope mounted, for distance use, on a bifocal lens.
B.   Telescopes mounted as binocular near spectacles.
Photos courtesy of Carl Zeiss.

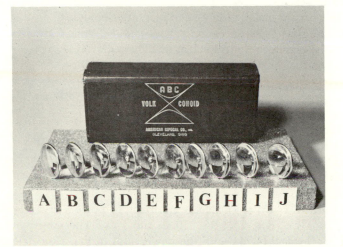

Fig. XIV-24. *Volk Conoid glass, aspheric, microscopic lenses. A. +15D.; B. +20D.; C. +25D.; D. +30D.; E. +35D.; F. +40D.; G. +50D.; H. +60D.; I. +80D.; J. +100D.*

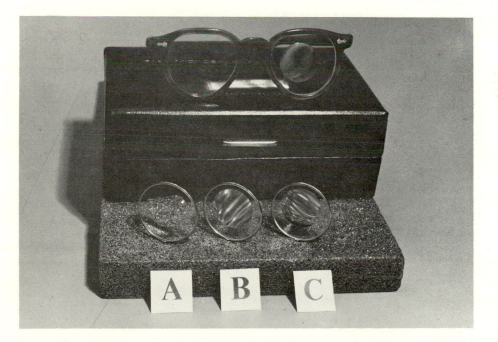

Fig. XIV-25. *American Optical glass bifocal microscopic lenses. A. 2X; B. 4X; C. 6X.*

corrections. Finished lenses are available in 40 mm. or 37 mm. diameters. For a small extra charge finished lenses can be ordered mounted in a hand magnifier holder.

ABC also has available glass aspheric cataract lenses called Volk Catraconoid Lenses. These are available in single vision or bifocal form in clear or light pink tint.

American Optical Company
A. American Optical produces the following types of lenses especially useful as microscopics:
1. Glass microscopic lenses
2. Aolite aspheric microscopic lenses
3. Aolite aspheric cataract lenses
4. Aolite high-add bifocal cataract lenses
5. Half-eye lenses in frames

B. Glass microscopic lenses

These lenses (see Figure XIV-25) are available normally in powers of 2×, 4×, 6×, and 8× and by special order in 1×, 3×, 5×, 7×, 9×, 10×, and 15×. The lenses are supplied in 54 mm. uncut or 81 mm. semi-finished blanks with the power spot in the geometric center, thus allowing incorporation of the distance Rx in the carrier portion and hence its use as a high-add bifocal. Because the carrier curve on the side of the power spot is plano, except the 2× which is ground on a +4.00D. base, (see Figure XIV-26), the lens is most useful where a plano or concave distance correction is required; otherwise, a poor lens form results for distance.

Because of blank thickness, there is a limit to the power of the distance Rx that can be supplied. The following specifications were supplied by American Optical Company through the courtesy of Mr. John Davis:

Magnification	Spot Diameter	Approximate Working Distance	Approximate Useful Field
2×	25 mm.	5 inches	4 ⅞ inches
4×	25 mm.	2 ½ inches	2 ¼ inches
6×	25 mm.	1 ⅝ inches	1 ⅜ inches
8×	25 mm.	1 ¼ inches	⅞ inches
Special Order			
1×-9× (odd powers)	25 mm.		
10×	15 mm.	1 inch	
15×	12 mm.	⅝ inch	

C. Aolite aspheric microscopic lenses

These lenses (see Figure XIV-27) are plastic aspheric supplied in specific powers of 6×, 8×, 10×, and 12× only. The lenses are available as 60 mm. uncuts with the spot diameter decreasing with increasing power. Because the lenses are cast, they are not available with any other prescription incorporated.

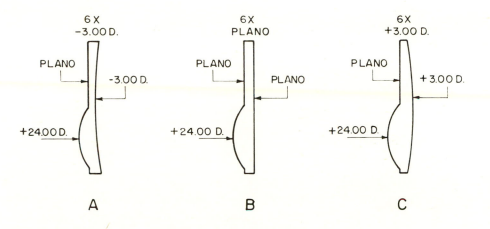

Fig. XIV-26.   *Line drawings in cross-section view of 6X American Optical glass bifocal microscopic lenses with power incorporated in the upper portion. It is apparent that the best lens forms result when the lenses are used with the microscopic segment on the front surface. Note in C, that a poor lens form (convex rear surface) results for the upper portion if the segment is on the front surface. If the lens is reversed so that the segment is on the rear surface, than a **very** poor lens form results for the microscopic portion.*

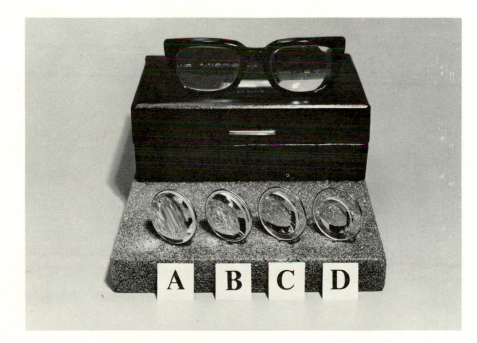

Fig. XIV-27.   *American Optical plastic, aspheric, microscopic lenses.*
A. 6x; B. 8x; C. 10X; D. 12X.

American Optical Company specifications are:

Magnification	Spot Diameter	Approximate Working Distance	Approximate Useful Field
6×	40 mm.	1 ⅜ inches	2 inches
8×	33 mm.	1 ⅛ inches	1 ⅜ inches
10×	29 mm.	⅞ inch	1 inch
12×	25 mm.	⅝ inch	¾ inch

D. Aolite aspheric cataract lenses

These lenses (see Figure XIV-28) are plastic aspheric lenses of higher powers designed as post-surgical cataract lenses. The lenses are available in both single vision and bifocal form and in clear or tinted. The base curves have been calculated based on distance vision requirements. However, John Davis (1971) of American Optical Company reports that his calculations show that, in the range of powers of the Aolite Aspheric Cataract lens, designing a special lens for near object distances offers insignificant advantages.

The lenses are available in powers +8.00 D. through +20.00 D. spherical powers and cylinder powers of –0.25 D. to –5.00 D. in 0.25 D. steps. It must be remembered that these powers are in terms of back focal length, while when used as microscopics, front focal length is the more significant measurement. Bifocal adds are +2.00 D., +2.50 D., +3.00 D., and +3.50 D. The power spot diameter is 40 mm. in all powers. The blank sizes are 56 mm. in diameter. The ocular curve is –3.77 D.

American Optical Company specifications are:

Back Focal Power	Magnification	Approximate Working Distance	Approximate Useful Field
+8.00	1.9×	5 ¼ inches	7 ⅛ inches
+9.00	2.1×	4 ⅝ inches	
+10.00	2.4×	4 ¼ inches	
+11.00	2.6×	3 ⅞ inches	
+12.00	2.8×	3 ⅝ inches	4 ¾ inches
+13.00	3.0×	3 ⅜ inches	
+14.00	3.2×	3 ⅛ inches	
+15.00	3.4×	3 inches	
+16.00	3.6×	2 ¾ inches	3 ⅝ inches
+17.00	3.8×	2 ⅝ inches	
+18.00	4.0×	2 ½ inches	
+19.00	4.1×	2 ½ inches	
+20.00	4.3×	2 ⅜ inches	2 ⅜ inches

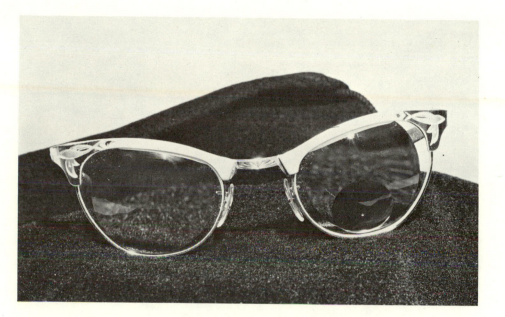

Fig. XIV-28. Plastic, lenticular, aspheric, cataract lenses.
Right eye: Single vision
Left eye: Bifocal

Plastic aspheric cataract lenses made by numerous other companies are available from local ophthalmic laboratories.

E. Aolite high-add bifocal cataract lenses

These lenses are plastic aspheric supplied in distance powers of +8.00 D. to +20.00 D. spheres with cylinder powers from –0.25D. through –5.00 D. in 0.25 D. cylinder steps. The adds are available in +6.00 D., +12.00 D., and +18.00 D. All lenses have a 40 mm. round power spot with a 22 mm. round segment on the front surface.

F. Half-eye lenses in frames

These aids (see Figure XIV-29) are plastic lenses finish mounted in zyl half-eye frames. Base-in prism is incorporated for binocular use.

The American Optical Company specifications are:

Back Focal Power	Base-in Prism
+6.00 D.	8 △ per lens
+8.00 D.	10 △ per lens
+10.00 D.	12 △ per lens

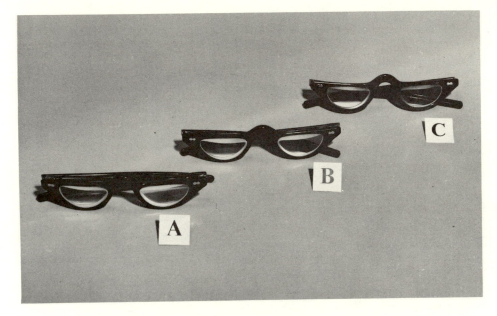

Fig. XIV-29. *American Optical plastic, prismatic, half-eye spectacles.*
    A.   + 6.00D. with 8 ^△ base-in per lens.
    B.   + 8.00D. with 10 ^△ base-in per lens.
    C.   + 10.00D. with 12 ^△ base-in per lens.

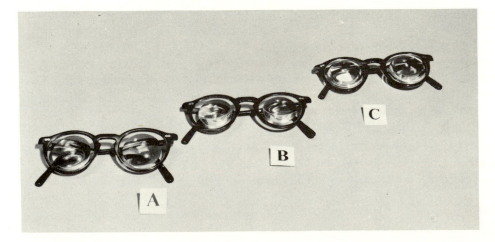

Fig. XIV-30. *Igard Hyperoculars; plastic, lenticular, aspheric, microscopic spectacles. Although the picture shows two lenses in each frame, there is no prism incorporated and thus they are for monocular use.*
    A. 6X; B. 8X; C. 10X.

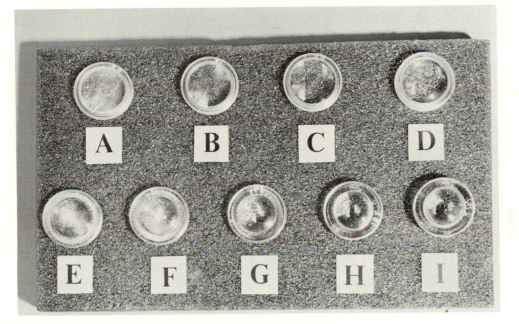

Fig. XIV-31. Feinbloom full field microscopic lenses.
A. 2X; B. 4X; C. 6X; D. 8X; E. 10X; F. 12X; G. 14X; H. 16X; I. 20X.

BSA Industries

BSA Industries manufactures a wide variety of CR-39 plastic lenses. Among these is a series of high add bifocals. The lenses are made with 25 mm. round segments located on the front surface of the lens. The blanks are 68 mm. round with the top of the segment 8 mm. below center.

These lenses are available in distance lens powers from −16.00 D. to +16.00 D. spheres combined with concave cylinders up to 4.00 D. Segment additions available are: +4.25; +4.50; +4.75; +5.00; +6.00; +7.00; +8.00; +9.00; +10.00 and +12.00 D.

Combined Optical Industries Ltd. (COIL)

COIL manufactures plastic aspheric microscopics under the name of Igard Hyperoculars (see Figures XIV-30). These lenses are available in powers of 4×, 6×, 8×, and 10×. They are biconvex with a lenticular flange resulting in an overall blank diameter of 49.6 mm. Cylindrical corrections cannot be incorporated.

Specifications are:

Magnification	Spot Diameter	Approximate Working Distance	Approximate Useful Field
4×	40.0 mm.	6.25 cm.	7.8 cm.
6×	36.0 mm.	4.16 cm.	5.5 cm.
8×	34.3 mm.	3.13 cm.	3.6 cm.
10×	40.0 mm.	2.50 cm.	1.9 cm.

Designs for Vision

Designs for Vision has available prescription microscopic lenses in full diameter, bifocal, and half-eye forms.

A. Full diameter microscopics

These lenses (see Figure XIV-31) are composed of glass airspaced doublet and triplet lenses mounted in plastic carriers. They are available in powers 2× through 20×. Cylindrical correction can be incorporated.

The standard prescription lenses are round. While the carrier may be edged to any shape, the minimum diameter in all meridians must be at least 38 mm. Thus, the frame must be at least 38 mm. in all eye size dimensions. Meredith Morgan (Morgan, 1972) has noted the following linear fields of fixation when the target is in the primary focal plane and the lens is as close to the eye as possible:

Magnification	Linear Field
2×	110 mm.
4×	68 mm.
6×	38 mm.
8×	28 mm.
10×	18 mm.
12×	17 mm.
14×	14 mm.
16×	11 mm.
20×	8 mm.

B. Bifocal microscopic lenses

These lenses (see Figure XIV-32) are insert type truncated oval segment bifocals supplied in two different segment sizes. The standard segment measures 13 mm. by 23 mm., while the Type R segment measures 17 mm. by 25 mm. A regular distance correction may be supplied in the plastic carrier lens with the microscopic power in the glass insert segment. The segment powers are available in 2× through 10×. Cylindrical corrections may be incorporated in the carrier or the segment or both.

Morgan (1972) has noted the linear field of the 4× Standard Segment to be 38 mm. when the target is in the primary focal plane of the lens.

The authors have measured the following:

Segment Type	Power	Linear Field Width
Standard	4×	38 mm.
Type R	2×	98 mm.
Type R	6×	41 mm.

C. Half-eye microscopic lenses

These lenses (see Figure XIV-33) are a glass-plastic combination similar to the full field made in a half-eye form. They are available in powers 2× through 10×.

The lens size is 23 mm. by 28 mm.

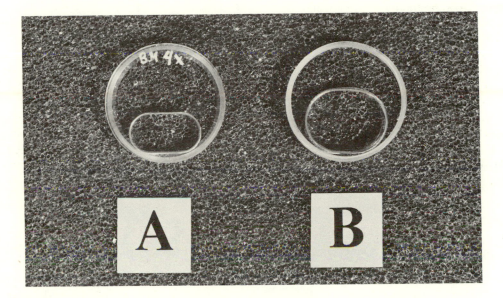

Fig. XIV-32.   *Feinbloom bifocal microscopic lenses.*
A.   *Standard 13 by 23 mm. segment.*
B.   *Type R 17 by 25 mm. segment.*

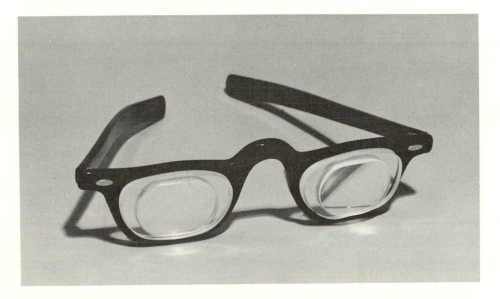

Fig. XIV-33.   *Feinbloom half-eye microscopic spectacles. Because prism is not incorporated, these spectacles are not designed for binocular use. One of the lenses is usually made as a dummy balance lens.*

Morgan (1972) has noted the following:

Magnification	Horizontal Field of Fixation
2×	120 mm.
6×	40 mm.
8×	33 mm.

Keeler Optical Products, Inc.

The following chart lists the microscopic spectacles manufactured by Keeler. The specifications are those of the manufacturer. All are fitted monocularly.

Keeler L.V.A. Number	Magnification	Form	Work Distance From Cornea (Cm.)	Object Field (Cm.)	Comments
L.V.A.9	8× 10× 12× 15× 20×	Full Field			Aspheric compound magnifier Focal distance maintainence housing with built-in illumination (or clear housing), battery or transformer. Also available as a stand magnifier. (See Figure XIV-34)
L.V.A. 10A	2× 3×	Full Field or Bifocal	13.5 9.5	12.0 9.0	Aspheric magnifier. Full field or Crescent shaped bifocal (See Figure XIV-35)
L.V.A.10B	4× 5× 6× 8×	Full Field or Bifocal	7.0 6.0 5.0 4.0	6.0 5.5 4.0 3.5	Aspheric magnifier. Full Field or Crescent shaped bifocal (See Figure XIV-35)
L.V.A.10C	6× 8×	Full Field	5.0 4.0	4.0 3.5	Aspheric magnifier. Incorporates a plastic focal distance maintaining piece (See Figure XIV-36)
L.V.A.12	2× 3× 4× 5× 6× 7× 8× 9×	Bifocal insert	13.5 9.5 7.0 6.0 5.0 4.5 4.0 3.5	8.0 5.0 4.5 4.5 3.0 3.0 2.5 2.0	Bifocal aspheric magnifier. Round plastic insert bifocal segment, threaded for interchangeability. (See Figure XIV-37)

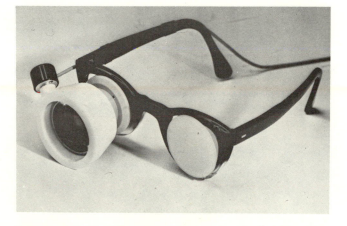

Fig. XIV-34. *Keeler monocular, full field, compound, aspheric, il-luminated, microscopic spectacles (L.V.A.-9). The illumination housing is adjustable for maintaining the object in focus. The power source for illumination, a battery handle, is not shown. Photo courtesy of Keeler Optical Products, Inc.*

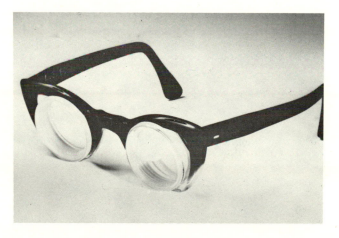

Fig. XIV-35. *Keeler monocular, aspheric, microscopic spectacles (L.V.A.-10A,B). Right eye: Full field. Left eye: Crescent shaped bifoc-al. Photo courtesy of Keeler Optical Products, Inc.*

Optical Sciences Group, Inc.

Optical Sciences Group manufactures Fresnel type flexible, vinyl, press-on prisms, and aspheric lenses which can be mounted on any spectacle lens to afford increased prismatic or refractive power without materially changing the lens thickness (see Figure XIV-38).

The refractive lenses and prisms are available as 63 mm. diameter round blanks. Certain of the refractive lenses are also available as pre-cut, 25 mm., "D" shaped segments. The D-segments

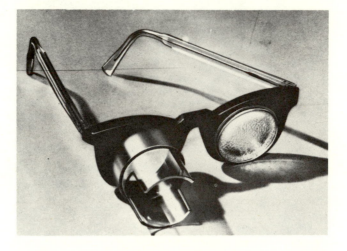

Fig. XIV-36.   Keeler monocular, aspheric, microscopic spectacles with plastic focal distance housing (L.V.A.-10C). Photo courtesy of Keeler Optical Products, Inc.

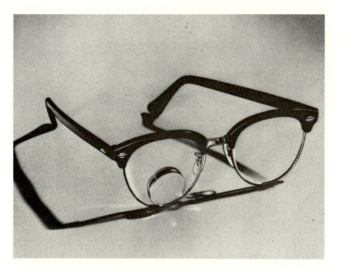

Fig. XIV-37.   Keeler monocular, plastic, aspheric, bifocal microscopic spectacles (L.V.A.-12). Photo courtesy of Keeler Optical Products, Inc.

are supplied in pairs of equal power. The D-segment lenses in powers +3.00 D. and above also contain a prismatic element to aid in maintenance of convergence when prescribed binocularly.

The present lens forms are designed to be mounted to the rear surface of the carrier spectacles.

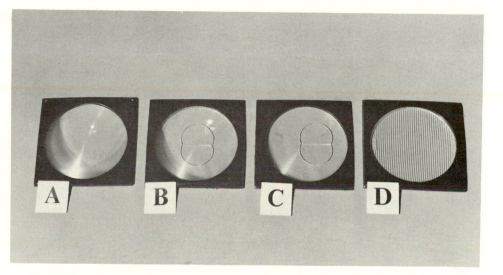

Fig. XIV-38.   O.S.G. Fresnel vinyl press-on lenses and prisms.
    A.   Convex lens.
    B.   D-shape bifocal segments.
    C.   D-shape bifocal segments with horizontal prism.
    D.   Plano prism.

Optical Sciences Group lists the following lenses available at this time:

Press-on Prisms   0.50 to 30 prism diopters

Press-on aspheric lenses (63 mm.)   +0.50 D. to +20.00 D. and –1.00 D. to –14.00 D.

Press-on D-25 Segments   Without prism control
                                  +0.50 D. to +2.50 D.

With prism control

Adds	Base-in Prism (per Seg)
+3.00 D.	1$^\triangle$
+3.50 D.	1.75$^\triangle$
+4.00 D.	2.5$^\triangle$
+5.00 D.	4$^\triangle$
+6.00 D.	5.5$^\triangle$
+7.00 D.	7$^\triangle$
+8.00 D.	8.5$^\triangle$

Policoff Laboratories

Policoff Laboratories manufactures a series of insert type bifocal microscopic lenses in add powers of 3×; 5×; 7×; 10×; and 14× (see Figure XIV-39). The 3× and 5× are cemented glass doublets, while the 7×, 10× and 14× are cemented glass triplets of Hastings design.

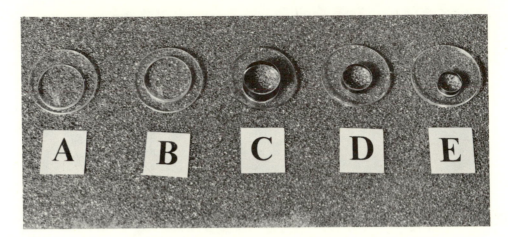

Fig. XIV-39.   Policoff insert, bifocal, microscopic lenses.
A. 3X; B. 5X; C. 7X; D. 10X; E. 14X.

The distance correction may be incorporated in the plastic carrier lens.

The segment shape in 3× and 5× may be round or D-shaped, while the 7×, 10× and 14× are only round. The segment size varies with the power.

Meredith Morgan (1972) has noted the following field parameters:

Magnification	Segment Diameter	Field of Fixation
3×	25 mm.	77 mm.
5×	25 mm.	44 mm.
7×	19 mm.	25 mm.
10×	15 mm.	11 mm.
14×	12 mm.	7 mm.

While the overall fields are small in the higher powers, it should be noted that the entire field is useable since they are clear from edge to edge.

Shuron-Continental

Shuron-Continental manufactures a series of high add ultex bifocals for low vision patients (see Figure XIV-40).

The lenses are available as 81 mm. round semi-finished blanks with the round power spot in the center of the blank. They are stocked at the factory, all on a –8.50 D. base. The segments are on the ocular surface.

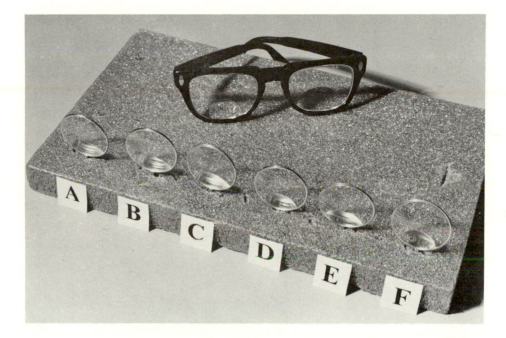

Fig. XIV-40.   Shuron-Continental high add ultex bifocal lenses.
Spectacles: Right eye: +20D.
Left eye: +5D.
A. +5D.; B. +6D.; C. +7D.; D. +10D.; E. +12D.; F. +20D.

They are available in the following additions:

Additional Power	Segment Size
+5.00 D.	32 mm.
+6.00 D.	32 mm.
+7.00 D.	32 mm.
+8.00 D.	32 mm.
+10.00 D.	26 mm.
+12.00 D.	26 mm.
+16.00 D.	22 mm.
+20.00 D.	22 mm.

These lenses should not be confused with the ordinary ultex bifocal which can be obtained in high powers on special order. The ordinary ultex blank size and segment location is much different and thus restricts the location of the segment in the finished spectacle.

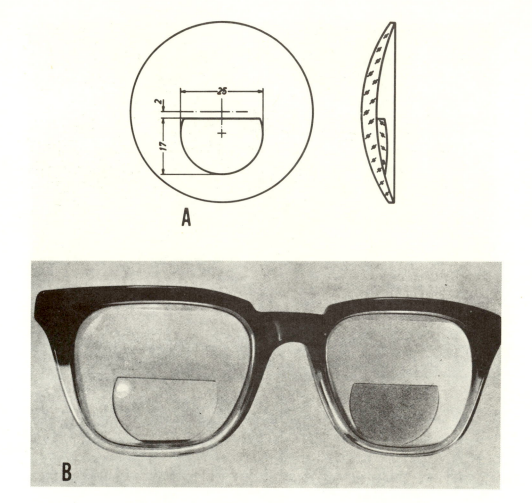

Fig. XIV-41.   *Zeiss glass, bifocal, microscopic spectacles. The bifocal segment is polymerized to the ocular surface of the carrier lens.*
   A.   Line drawings.
   B.   Spectacles showing the right lens, a microscopic segment, and the left lens, an occluder segment.
   Photos courtesy of Carl Zeiss.

Zeiss

Carl Zeiss manufactures an all-glass bifocal microscopic in additions of 2×; 3×; and 4×. The segment is a flat top type, measuring 17 mm. by 25 mm., and is located on the ocular surface of the carrier lens (see Figure XIV-41). Distance corrections can be incorporated in the carrier lens, but are available only in 1.00 D. steps except by special order.

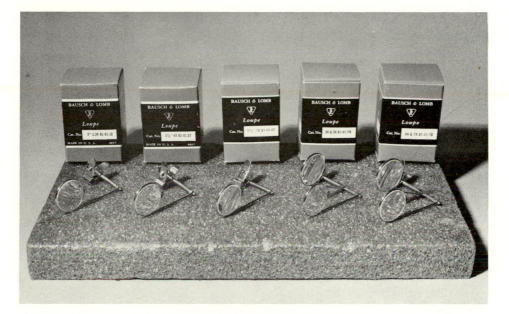

Fig. XIV-42.   B. & L. eyeglass loupes.

Loupes

Loupes and Lenses, Clip-On

A. Bausch & Lomb

Bausch & Lomb eyeglass loupes (see Figure XIV-42) consist of one or more 25 mm. diameter biconvex lenses mounted in a gold finished metal holder which attaches to eyeglass temples and can easily be flipped out of the line of sight.

Bausch & Lomb lists the following specifications:

Magnification	Working Distance
3×	3.3 inches
3.3×	3 inches
4×	2.5 inches
5×	2 inches
7×	1.5 inches
4, 7×	2.5, 1.5 inches
3, 5×	3.3, 2 inches

Similar loupes with a different attachment clip are available also from the Behr Manufacturing Company.

B. The Lighthouse (New York Association For The Blind)

Ary loupes, opaque sided, flip-up, clip-on devices (see Figure XIV-43) are available in 1-inch

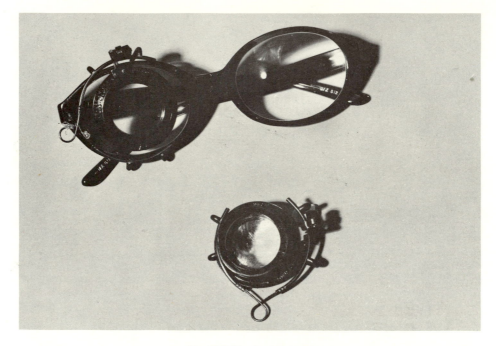

Fig. XIV-43.   Ary loupes.

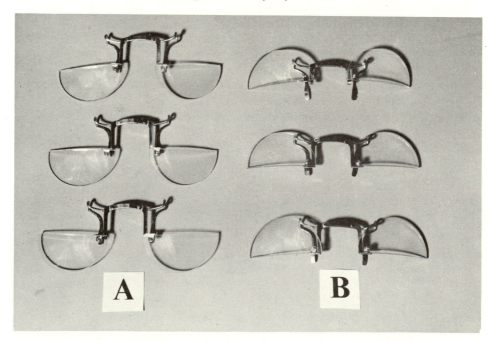

Fig. XIV-44.   Clip-on bifocals in powers +1.25D.; +2.00D.; and +3.00D.
  A.   Magna-Adds.
  B.   Magna-U's.

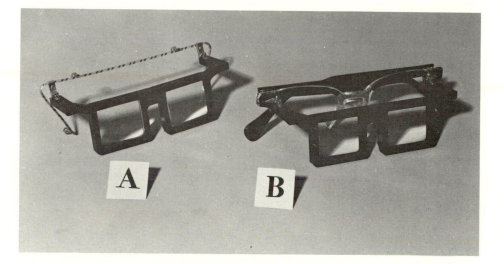

Fig. XIV-45. Telesight flip-up binocular loupes.
A. Clip-on.
B. Loupe permanently attached to a half frame.

diameter lenses in the following powers: +10.00 D., +11.00 D., +12.00 D., +16.00 D., +20.00 D., +25.00 D., and +32.00 D.

C. Magna-Add

Magna-Add manufactures clip-on plastic ½-lenses in two forms. The Magna-Add form places the added lens on the lower section of the eyeglass lens while the Magnu-U form places the added lens on the upper section of the eyeglass lens (see Figure XIV-44). Either form is available with lens powers of +1.25 D., +2.00 D., and +3.00 D. One may also obtain the mountings alone, if one desires to substitute lenses of other powers.

D. Telesight

Telesight has binocular loupes which can be ordered as clip-on units or attached to half or full frames (see Figure XIV-45). Telesight lists the focal lengths available as: 20″; 13⅓″; 10″; 8″; 6⅔″; 5″; 4½″; and 4″. An extra lens is available which can be attached to the front of the loupes which swings out of the way when not needed. Telesight lists this as adding 2½×.

Telesight also supplies a clip-on, flip-up, aspheric plastic lens in lenticular form which is available in powers of +16.00 D., +24.00 D., and +32.00 D. The lenses used are the COIL Igard Hyperoculars discussed under Microscopics in this chapter.

Loupes, Headborne

A. Bausch & Lomb

Bausch & Lomb manufactures a headband binocular loupe called the Magna-Visor (see Figure XIV-46). Bausch & Lomb lists the powers as 1½×, 2¼×, and 3½×. The lenses are plastic and are available separately as extra or replacement lenses. An auxiliary lens is also available which mounts centrally on the front of the visor and then can be located in front of either eye.

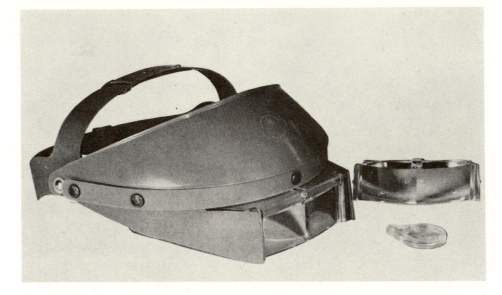

Fib. XIV-46.   B. & L. Magna-Visor binocular loupe. Also shown is an extra insert of a different power as well as a monocular auxiliary lens.

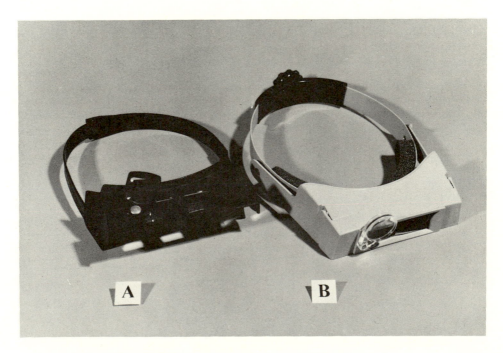

Fig. XIV-47.   Edroy Magni-focuser binocular loupes.
   A.   Mark I.
   B.   Mark II.

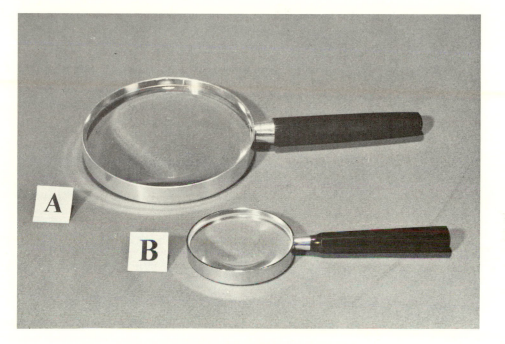

Fig. XIV-48.   Hand held magnifiers.
A.   +4.00D., 4-½" diameter.
B.   +6.50D., 2-½" diameter.

The visor is equipped with an over-eye visor, side shields, and sweat band, all of which can be removed for cleaning or if not needed. In addition to the usual band which fits around the head, the visor is equipped with an over-the-head band which helps steady the device.

B. Edroy
Edroy distributes the headborne binocular loupe called Magni-focuser (see Figure XIV-47). It is available with lenses with focal lengths of 20", 14", 8", 6", and 4". An auxilliary lens is available for the 14", 8", and 6" models which can be attached to swing in front of one eye which then affords total focal lengths of 4", 3", and 2", respectively.
This device is available also through several other distributors; such as Apex and New Era.
Other devices similar to the Magna-Visor or the Magni-focuser are available from many other distributors such as: Bernell Corporation, Donegan Optical Company, House of Vision, New Era Optical Company, and others.

Magnifiers
The number of magnifiers and their sources is incalculable. Thus, only representative types will be discussed here. The omission of a particular one or type does not imply that it is any less useful.

Hand Held
The venerable biconvex lens mounted in a metal ring with a black handle is still the most frequently used and mostly self-prescribed low vision aid (see Figure XIV-48). Large selections of

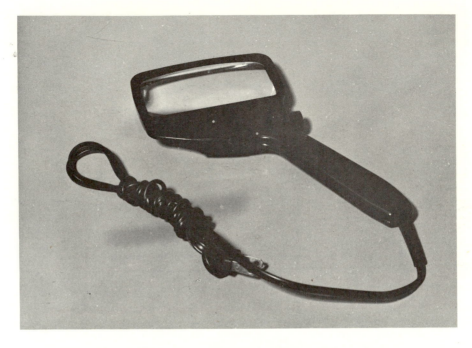

Fig. XIV-49.   B. & L. illuminated Rectangular Reader, + 4.50D.

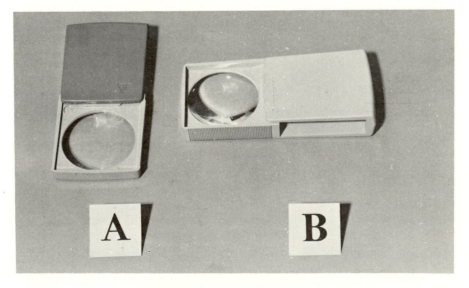

Fig. XIV-50.   B. & L. Packette Magnifiers.
A.   3X.
B.   5X.

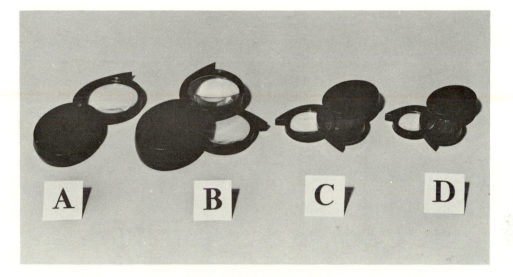

Fig. XIV-51.   Folding pocket magnifiers.
A.   3X; 35mm. diameter.
B.   3X, 4X, 7X; 35mm. diameter.
C.   4X, 5X, 9X; 23mm. diameter.
D.   5X, 7X, 12X; 20mm. diameter.

these and other hand magnifiers are available from Apex Specialties, Colonial Optical, New Era, Prentiss, Selsi, Swift, and many others.

A. Bausch & Lomb

Bausch & Lomb manufactures several different hand held magnifiers. Some of these require special mention.

   1. The Rectangular Reader is a lens measuring 3⅞″ by 2″ with a 9″ focus, mounted in a rectangular shaped holder with an attached handle (see Figure XIV-49). This device is available with or without built-in illumination.

   2. Pocket magnifiers

      a. The Packette Magnifier is composed of a 3× or 5×, 35 mm. diameter lens mounted in a square, hard plastic holder which slides into an attached hard plastic housing when not in use (see Figure XIV-50).

      b. Two round lens magnifiers are available which fold into an attached vinyl-like case when not in use. Both lenses are mounted in a plastic ring. The 1½″ diameter lens is 2× and swings into a square case. The 2″ diameter lens is 2× and swings into a semi-round case (see Figure XIV-57).

      c. Folding pocket magnifiers are a series of lenses of various diameters and powers mounted in a hard plastic ring which swings into a hard plastic housing when not in use (see Figure XIV-51). These devices are available with single, double, or triple lenses attached to the same housing. Powers and combinations are available from 3× to 20× with lens diameters from 35 mm. to 17 mm.

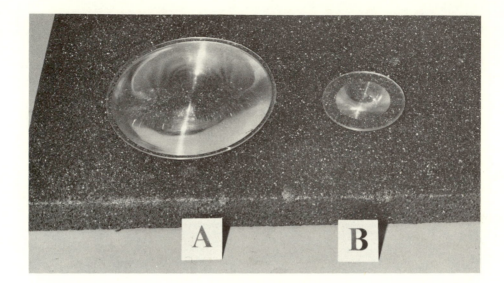

Fig. XIV-52   Bolsey Fresnel lenses.
A.   + 14.50D., 4″ diameter.
B.   + 47.00D., 1.3″ diameter.

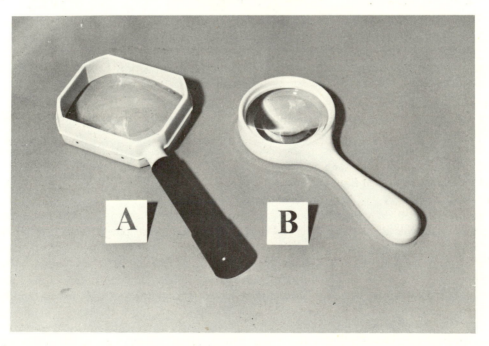

Fig. XIV-53.   COIL plastic, aspheric, hand held magnifiers.
A.   + 11.50D., 2-¾″ by 2-¼″ (S-432).
B. + 20.00D., 53mm. diameter (S-460).

B. Bolsey Research and Development

Bolsey manufactures hard plastic Fresnel principle lenses, some of which can be used as hand magnifiers (see Figure XIV-52). The following are of special interest:

Size	Thickness	Focal Length
1 ½″ × 4″	.020″	2.75″
1.3″ diameter	.050″	0.850″
4″ diameter	.050″ or .020″	2.78″
10″ diameter	.080″	8″
11″ diameter	.080″	12.5″
15″ diameter	.080″	12.5″

C. Combined Optical Industries Limited (COIL)

This company manufactures many hand held plastic magnifiers, both spheric and aspheric in form (see Figure XIV-53). Some of the more frequently used are:

Name	Power	Lens Size
S-5247 Handmagnifier	+12.00 D.	2″ diameter
S-482 Welterweight	+4.00 D.	3 ½″ by 2 ½″
S-1014 Empress	+5.00 D.	2 ½″ by 1 ¾″
S-478 Flyweight	+6.00 D.	2 ⅛″ by 1 ½″
Aspherics		
S-449 Major Reader	+6.00 D.	4″ by 3″
S-442 Large Hand Reader	+8.00 D.	4″ by 3″
S-432 Small Hand Reader	+11.50 D.	2 ¾″ by 2 ¼″
S-460 Cataract Hand Reader	+20.00 D.	53 mm. diameter

Most of these COIL magnifiers are available in the United States from Donegan, Edroy, the N. Y. Lighthouse, McLeod, Telesight, and others.

D. Edmunds Scientific

Edmunds Scientific has listed a "Fresnel Burning Lens" (see Figure XIV-54). This is a hard plastic +5.50 D. Fresnel lens which measures 2-3/16″ by 3½″. Located in one corner there is an 11/16″ diameter +22.00 D. biconvex lens area of greater power.

E. Electro-Optix, Inc.

This company manufactures the Pathfinder which is a self-illuminating hand held magnifier whose over-all size is 53 mm. square by 20 mm. thick (see Figure XIV-55). It is available with a lens of either +16.00 D. or +32.00 D. which measures 25 mm. in diameter. The small bulb which is angled so as to project light on the field of the lens is powered by two AAA size penlight batteries. The device is available in several different colors and comes equipped with a soft vinyl snap-lock pouch. A similar illuminated magnifier with a plastic housing instead of metal is available from Electro-Optix under the name Scanner.

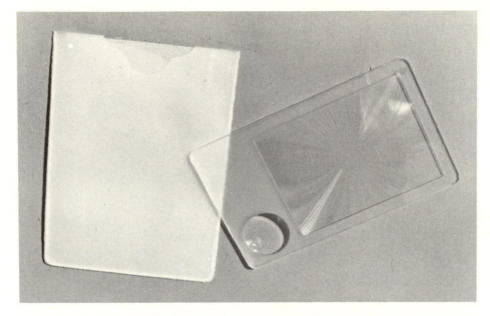

Fig. XIV-54.   Fresnel Burning Lens and case.

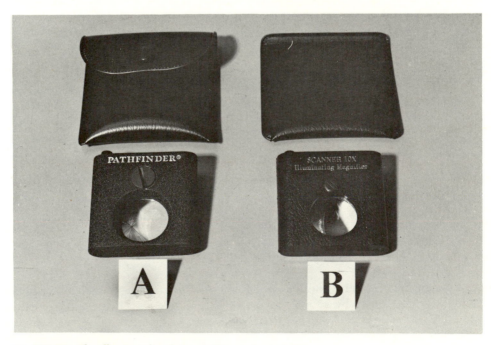

Fig. XIV-55.   Flex illuminated pocket magnifiers and carrying cases.
   A.   Pathfinder, +16.00D.
   B.   Scanner, +32.00D.
   The Pathfinder consists of a glass lens mounted in a metal housing, while the Scanner is made with a plastic lens and a plastic housing. Both models are available in the two powers.

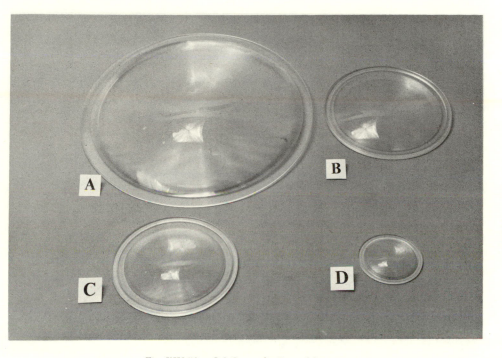

Fig. XIV-56.   O.S.G. acrylic Fresnel lenses.
   A.   + 5.00D.; 10″ diameter.
   B.   + 5.50D.; 5″ diameter.
   C.   + 10.00D.; 4″ diameter.
   D.   + 20.00D.; 2″ diameter.

F. Optical Sciences Group

Optical Sciences Group manufactures several hard plastic (acrylic) Fresnel principle lenses which can be used as hand held magnifiers (see Figure XIV-56). Those currently available are:

Focal Length	Lens Diameter
+ 5.00 D.	10″
+ 5.50 D.	5″
+ 10.00 D.	4″
+ 14.00 D.	4″
+ 20.00 D.	2″
+ 39.00 D.	1″

When these lenses are held some distance away from the spectacle plane, the smooth surface should be placed away from the eye. When the lenses are held near the spectacle plane, the smooth surface should be placed toward the eye. The lenses have no handles but do have a small raised rim to protect the grooves.

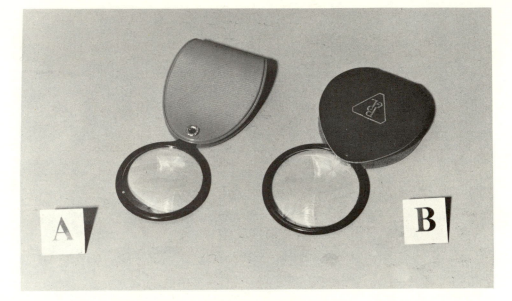

Fig. XIV-57.   Pocket magnifiers.
A.   Selsi: +11.25D.; 1 ¾'' diameter.
B.   B & L.: +8.00D.; 2'' diameter.

G. Selsi

1. Selsi supplies various round magnifiers with an attached vinyl-like case (see Figure XIV-57). The lenses are usually 1¾ inches in diameter and +11.00 D. in power. These are also available from the N. Y. Lighthouse which also carries a similar one listed as number 424 which is +16.00 D. vertex power.

2. Selsi also supplies a neck-held magnifier. A 4 inch diameter lens of +4.00 D. is mounted in a plastic frame which rests on the user's chest. An attached cord fits around the user's neck to hold the magnifier in place (see Figure XIV-58). This device may also be used as a hand magnifier.

Stand Magnifiers

Stand Magnifiers are available from many sources. Only representative types of those most frequently used will be discussed here.

A. Focusable

1. Apex Specialties

The Gooseneck type of magnifier (see Figure XIV-59) is available in many powers and lens sizes from several suppliers. Apex lists the following specifications in their catalogue:

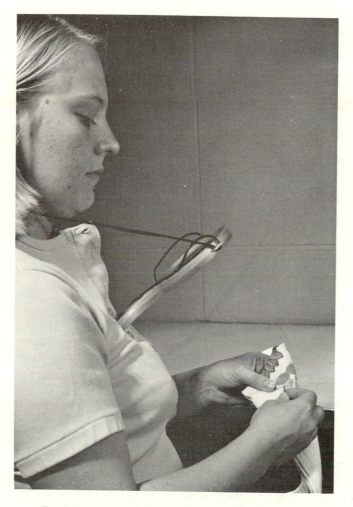

Fig. XIV-58.   Neck-held magnifier; +4.00D., 4″ diameter.

Lens Diameter	*Power*
3½″	+5.00 D.
4″	+4.00 D.
4½″	+3.50 D.
5″	+3.00 D.
2″ by 4″	+5.00 D.

The devices are available with or without attached illumination.

2. The N. Y. Lighthouse

The Lighthouse supplies Sloan focusable stand magnifiers as well as their attachments (see

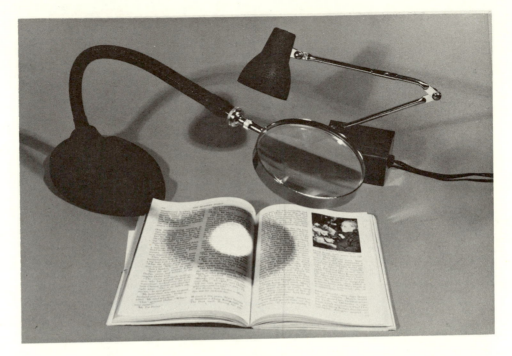

Fig. XIV-59.   Gooseneck stand magnifier; +4.00D., 4″ diameter.

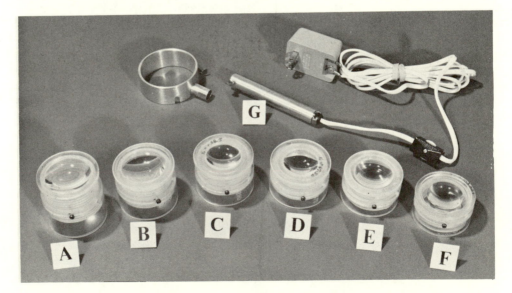

Fig. XIV-60. Sloan focusable stand magnifiers and illuminating handle.
A.   +18D.; B.   +23D.; C.   +29D.; D.   +37D.; E.   +44D.; F. +53D.; G. Illuminating handle, AC.

Figure XIV-60). These magnifiers are composed of lenses mounted in a clear plastic, externally threaded housing. This housing fits into an internally threaded clear plastic collar (stand). By screwing the lens housing in or out of the collar, the distance from the lens to the end of the collar (the object distance) may be varied.

115-Volt AC metal illuminator holders are available into which these stands fit where self-illumination is desired.

The housings are marked with the *Equivalent* power of the lenses and those available are listed in the following table. The authors have estimated the front vertex power for each magnifier and these specifications are also included.

Lens Size	Equivalent Power	Estimated Front Vertex Power
1½″	+18 D.	+18 D.
1½″	+23 D.	+24.5 D.
1¼″	+29 D.	+38.5 D.
1⅛″	+37 D.	+47.5 D.
1½″	+44 D.	+65 D.
1⅜″	+53 D.	+100 D.

B. Non-focusable

1. Combined Optical Industries Limited (COIL)

COIL manufactures non-focusable stand magnifiers in several powers. The plastic lenses are either rectangular or round in shape and are mounted in stands that readily allow for good illumination of the object to be viewed (see Figure XIV-61). In all of these magnifiers, the stand height is less than the ordinary focal distance of the lens. Thus, if the eye is held too close to the lens an added plus lens will be necessary for an emmetrope to see clearly without accommodation. These devices are usually used in a manner in which the distance from the eye to the lens is adjusted by the user so that the material viewed is in clear focus. COIL lists the following specifications for their aspheric stand magnifiers:

Name	Power	Lens Size
S-569 The Monarch	+ 4.50 D.	6½″ × 4⅛″
S-472 Large Stand	+ 8.00 D.	4″ × 3″
S-474 Small Stand	+11.50 D.	2¾″ × 2¼″
S-428 Cataract Stand	+20.00 D.	50 mm. diameter
S-1023 Hi-Power	+29.00 D.	38 mm. diameter

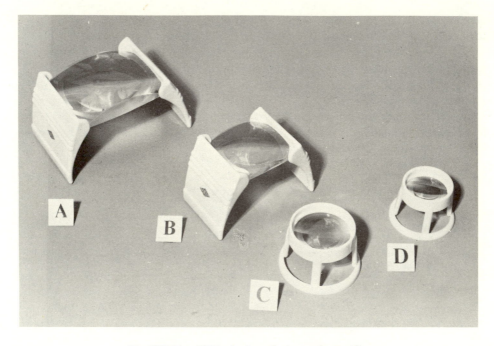

Fig. XIV-61.   COIL plastic aspheric stand magnifiers.
  A.   + 8.00D., 4″ by 3″ (S-472).
  B.   +11.50D., 2-¾″ by 2-¼″ (S-474).
  C.   +20.00D., 50mm. diameter (S-428).
  D.   +29.00D., 38mm. diameter (S-1023).

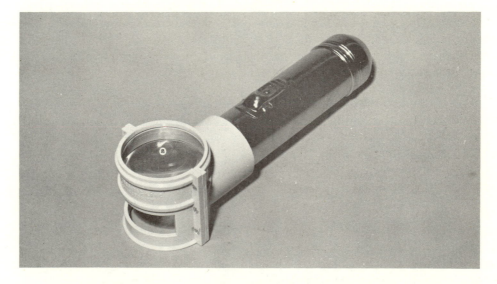

Fig. XIV-62.   Adisco illuminated magnifier; 5×, 47mm. diameter.

Most of these magnifiers are available in the United States from Donegan, Edroy, The N. Y. Lighthouse, McLeod, Telesight, and others.

2. The N. Y. Lighthouse

The Lighthouse has available the Adisco illuminated (flashlight) magnifier (see Figure XIV-62). This magnifier is rated at 5×. When material is placed against the front of the lens housing, it is inside the front focal plane of the lens system. Thus, material placed against the front of the housing will not be in focus for the emmetrope without the use of accommodation or a reading addition. This device is best used when held in the spectacle plane rather than in the usual position of hand or stand magnifiers. When used in this manner, not only is the field of view increased but aberrations are minimally effective.

This device is also available from Covington Plating Works in the battery model or in a 110-Volt AC model.

3. Selsi

Selsi lists several different stand magnifiers, both focusable and non-focusable. Three non-focusable stand magnifiers merit special comment here because of their frequency of use. These are the flashlight handle illuminated magnifiers (see Figure XIV-63). These devices are available through many other distributors, but all are similar. Selsi's specifications are:

Power	Ocular Lens Diameter	Battery Size
5×	47 mm.	D
7×	30 mm.	C
10×	30 mm.	C

With all three of these devices, the front of the housing is somewhat nearer the front focal plane of the lens system. In order to afford the largest possible field and minimize the aberration effects, these devices are best located with the ocular lens near the spectacle plane. Thus, if the devices are to be used this way and the material is to be held against the front of the housing, approximately a +4.00 D. lens must be held between the eye and the magnifier for the material to be in best focus for an emmetrope without using accommodation.

Another stand magnifier available from Selsi is the so-called "dome" magnifier (see Figure XIV-64). This magnifier is a thick, plano-convex lens. The authors measured the following specifications:

Rim	Center Thickness	Edge Thickness	Lens Diameter	Magnification
Chrome plated	34 mm.	20 mm.	60 mm.	1.5×

The same magnifier is also available from the N. Y. Lighthouse.

Since this device is usually used with the lens resting on the material to be magnified, the material is within the primary focal plane and, thus, accommodation or a reading addition will be required for an emmetrope.

Although "dome" magnifiers usually afford low magnification, they possess two distinct

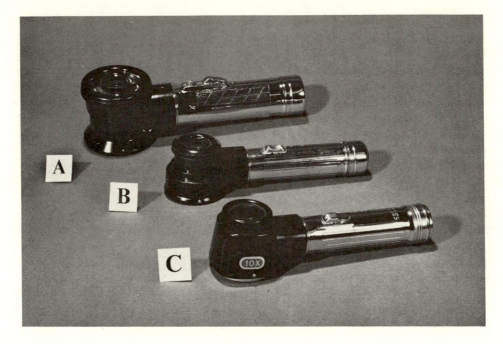

Fig. XIV-63.   Illuminated (flashlight) magnifiers.
A.   5X, 47mm. diameter.
B.   7X, 30 mm. diameter.
C.   10X, 30mm. diameter.

advantages. Unlike most other stand magnifiers, it is not necessary for the line of sight to be perpendicular to lens surface at its pole. They also exhibit very good light gathering properties.
4. Visolette
Visolette magnifiers are "dome" type stand magnifiers which are available in several sizes (see **Figure XIV-65**). The following are those available from Dr. Marvin Efron:

Rim	Lens Diameter	Magnification
Plastic	28 mm.	1.7×
	39 mm.	1.7×
	60 mm.	1.7×
Rubber	75 mm.	1.7×
	90 mm.	1.7×

The 60 mm. also is available with a 20 mm. round bifocal segment which affords 2.5× magnification. The Visolettes are also available from Designs for Vision.

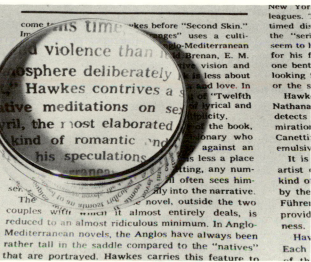

Fig. XIV-64.   Selsi dome stand magnifier; 1.5X, 60mm. diameter.

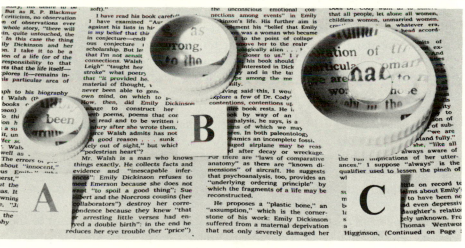

Fig. XIV-65.   Visolette dome stand magnifier.
    A.   1.7X, 28mm. diameter.
    B.   1.7X, 39mm. diameter.
    C.   1.7X, 60mm. diameter with bifocal segment 2.5X, 20mm. diame-
ter.

Projection Magnifiers

Optical Projection Magnifiers

A. Optiscope Enlarger

The Optiscope Enlarger is an opaque type projector which is available from Opaque Systems, Ltd. (see Figure XIV-66). The manufacturer's specifications are:

Magnification: 4×
Screen size: 9″ × 14″
Dimensions: 16″W × 17″H × 20¼″D
Weight: 14 lbs.

Electronic Projection Magnifiers

Ever since Dr. Samuel Genensky at Rand Corporation designed and publicized a closed circuit television system as a low vision aid, there has been much interest throughout the low vision field in the utilization of this type of device (see Figure V-8). There has been a proliferation of manufacturers and designs in the short time since the first commercial model was produced. This proliferation is still going on at such a rapid pace that any descriptions of specific manufacturers' models would be obsolete by the time this material is published. All of these devices do have certain elements in common and those elements will be discussed here. The advantages of any one design over any other will be omitted for fear of obsolescence.

All of the closed circuit television systems are composed of a television camera which is connected to a television monitor. The camera may be equipped with different fixed power lenses or with a zoom lens which will allow the user to vary the magnification. The systems are focusable to allow for various thicknesses of material. Some designs allow the camera to focus directly on the materials, while others focus the camera on the material by way of a mirror. The devices are usually available with different size monitors, or arrangements can be made to connect to a home television system. The monitors all allow for brightness control as well as the reverse polarity (changing black print on white background to white on black). Some devices are capable of better picture quality than others even where quality of components is equal due to a greater number of lines of resolution.

The devices usually come with an X-Y table, either built-in or separate, which allows for easy movement of the material. Some devices have a built-in illumination source for illuminating the material. Others require a separate illumination source. Typewriter attachments are presently available for some models. It is expected that in time other attachments will be designed and made available to meet other needs.

The major suppliers of closed circuit television systems for low vision known to the authors at the present time are: Apollo Laser, Designs for Vision, Opaque Systems Ltd., Pelco Sales Inc., Visualtek, and X/pert. There are a number of others which are less well known at this time.

Illumination Controls

Typoscopes

A. Designs for Vision

Designs for Vision supplies typoscopes which measure 5 inches wide by 3½ inches high. The vertically decentered viewing slot measures 4 inches wide by 7/16 inches high (see Figure VII-12). This typoscope is made of a thin, black, somewhat flexible, plastic material which can be wiped off when soiled.

B. Superior Optical Company

Superior Optical Company's typoscope is somewhat thicker and less flexible than the Designs for

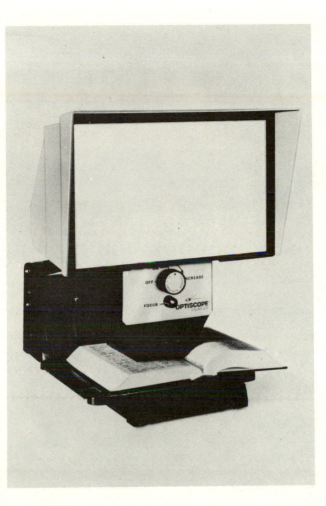

Fig. XIV-66. *Optiscope enlarger. Photo courtesy of Opaque Systems, Ltd.*

Vision model and is made of porous, fiberboard-like material (see Figure XIV-67). The overall size is 7 inches wide by 2¼ inches high with a horizontally decentered viewing slot measuring 4¼ inches wide by ⅜ inch high.

Visors, Side Shields, and Pin Holes
A. Eberson Enterprises
Eberson Enterprises supplies a "Sports Visor" which attaches to spectacles by two vinyl sleeves through which the temples slide (see Figure XIV-68). It is available in several colors besides black as well as a transparent green. This visor measures 7 inches wide by 3 inches deep.

B. Kono Manufacturing Company
In their Rare Visual Aids Catalogue, Kono lists both stationary and moveable side shields as well as

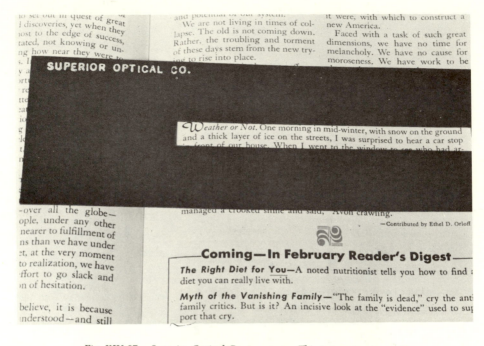

Fig. XIV-67.   Superior Optical Co. typoscope. This typoscope was patterned by Russell Stimson according to the original specifications given by Charles Prentice.

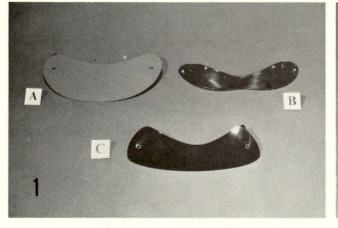
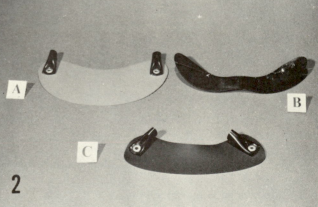

Fig. XIV-68.   Visors.
   A.   Eberson Sports Visor.
   B.   Nu-Vue Visor.
   C.   Visorette.
   View:
   1.   Top
   2.   Bottom, showing means of attachment to spectacles.

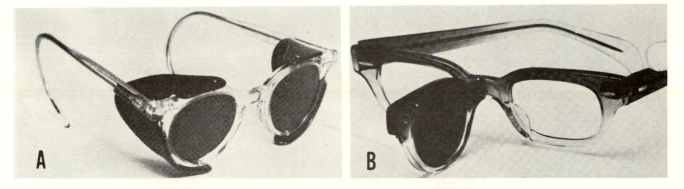

Fig. XIV-69.   A. Folding side shields.
B.   Kono swinging occluder.
Photo courtesy of Kono Manufacturing Co.

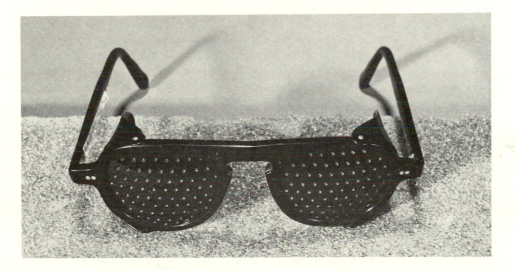

Fig. XIV-70.   May multiple pinhole spectacles with folding side shields.

a swinging occluder (see Figure XIV-69). These devices must be ordered through the local ophthalmic laboratory as Kono does not deal directly with the practitioner.

C. May Manufacturing Company

May Manufacturing Company has available single or multiple pinhole spectacles with attached opaque side shields (see Figure XIV-70). The plastic frames are supplied in 46 mm. eye size with 22 mm. or 24 mm. bridges. They also will supply a blank black disc for occlusion or designing a stenopaic slit.

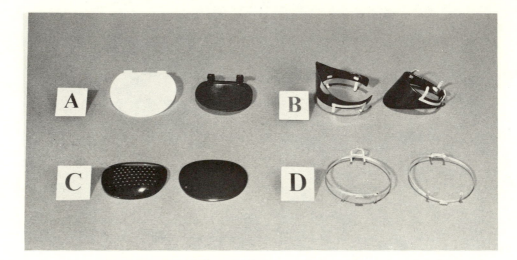

Fig. XIV-71.   Watchemoket ancillary aids.
  A.   Opaque clip-on occluders.
  B.   Opaque clip-on side shields.
  C.   Multiple pinhole and occluder discs to fit spectacle eyewires.
  D.   Monocular, spring-loaded, clip-on frames.

D. Nu-Vue Visor Company

This visor measures 7 inches wide and extends approximately 1¼ inches in front of each eye (see Figure XIV-68). It attaches to spectacles by two elastic bands which fit around the spectacle temples. The visor is available in black and brown, both of which are opaque.

E. Visorette

The Visorette attaches to spectacles by means of vinyl sleeves through which the spectacle temples slide (see Figure XIV-68). It measures 6½ inches wide by 1¾ inches deep. The visor is available in opaque black or transparent green with any one of four sizes of connector tubes.
The black visor is also available from The New York Lighthouse.

F. Watchemoket Optical Company, Inc.

Watchemoket supplies various occluders, side shields, and multiple pinhole discs (see Figure XIV-71). Occluders are available as snap-in types which can be mounted in spectacle frames or as clip-ons. The clip-on occluders are available with or without side shields.
The multiple pinhole is supplied as a disc only, however, Watchemoket also has available a monocular metal wire rim clip-on into which discs can be mounted.
Side shields are supplied in clip-on form only.
All of the above devices are available in various sizes and colors as well as round or P-3 shapes.

Tinted Lenses

Clip-on type, high quality sunglasses with glass or plastic lenses are available from many of the regular ophthalmic sunglass manufacturers such as American Optical Company, Bausch & Lomb, Victory Optical Company, and others.

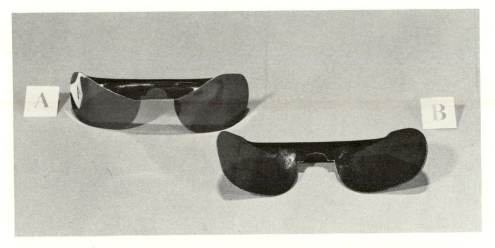

Fig. XIV-72.   Yorktown slip-in sun shades.
A.   Front view of grey tinted.
B.   Back view of green tinted.

Any optical low vision device from which the lenses can be removed can have color added to the lenses either through optical coatings or plastic dyes. In the case of devices incorporating a tube (telescopes), a tinted lens may be added to the device by having the lens mounted into the proper size camera filter holder and then attaching this to the aid.

A. Yorktowne Optical Company

Yorktowne Optical Company has available a wrap-around, slip-in celluloid sun shade which attaches to spectacle frames, fitting between the spectacles and the eyes (see Figure XIV-72). The shade includes a portion that wraps around as a side shield. The device is available in both grey and green. The authors have found that the grey transmits 25% and the green 20% across the visible spectrum. In the ultra-violet region, the grey transmits 8% and the green transmits less than 1%.

Lamps

Lamps are made in countless designs and are available from many sources too numerous to list here. Local stationary suppliers and lamp stores usually stock a variety of types. High intensity lamps have become very popular with low vision practitioners in recent times, probably because of their compactness and ease of directing the light (see Figure IX-3A). Some of these also have the advantage of minimizing heat radiance for very short working distances when the lamp may be located very close to the face. Perhaps the best known high intensity lamps are the Tensor series, however, many, many others are available.

Where a floor stand lamp is more practical, the goose neck lamps available through surgical supply stores are very useful (see Figure IX-3B). These are especially advantageous, where the light source needs to be very close to the material being viewed, because of their great adjustability.

Chapter 15

Non-Optical Aids

Introduction

Generally, optometrists and ophthalmologists underemphasize the use of non-optical aids while laymen are apt to overemphasize their use for the partially-sighted. Either attitude may be economically wasteful. Too often, the person advising a partially-sighted patient has a restricted field of thinking and scotomas in knowledge resulting in advising and prescribing devices with which he is most familiar, rather than devices that will produce the best results for the patient.

Sometimes doctors have learned the rules so well they have forgotten the exceptions. Experience with the presbyope who takes a telephone book out in the bright sunlight has taught us that it is easier and better to prescribe convex lenses to solve this problem. We then apply this same lesson to a person with macular degeneration and think that a +20 diopter add is preferable to increased illumination; or even worse, that the patient who cannot read in normal illumination with a normal add, cannot read.

Types of Aids

Illumination Control Devices

This very important classification is discussed in Chapter IX—Illumination.

Non-optical Magnification

A. Large print books

1. Large print makes use of the principle of relative size magnification (see Chapter V—Magnification) and has been widely used by educators in special books for school children. In recent years large print books for adults as well as special editions of newspapers (*New York Times*) and magazines (*Reader's Digest*) have been made available (see Figure XV-1).

2. Fonda (1965) has emphasized the point that large print books have too often been used where regular size type could easily have been used by the same student holding the book closer, perhaps with the aid of lenses.

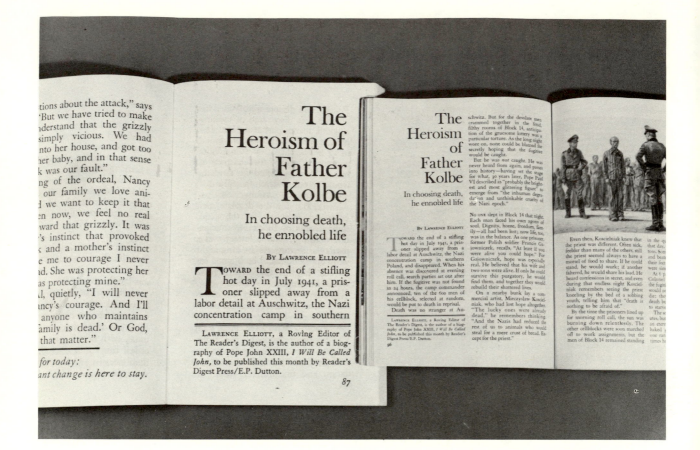

Fig. XV-1. Large print Reader's Digest compared to the standard edition. The 18 point (lower case 2.15M) type of the large print edition is twice the size of that of the standard edition. The publishers have taken special care in designing this large print edition to keep the book size closer to the standard edition than is usually the case with large print publications. To accomplish this, a quantity of material, including all advertisements have been eliminated. (Reproduced by permission of The Reader's Digest Association).

3. The cost of large print books in special editions, their increased size, and their limited availability makes this a very economically and educationally wasteful substitute for a low vision aid.

4. In teaching the mechanics of reading it may be more advantageous to use large print without the complications of closer working distances, optical aids, and special illumination. The hazard that must be avoided is the continued use and total dependence upon large print beyond the point where it is more advantageous than regular size type used with optical aids.

5. Where acuity is very poor and very high orders of magnification are required, a combination of an optical aid which permits relative distance magnification and large print which provides relative size magnification may be the preferred solution.

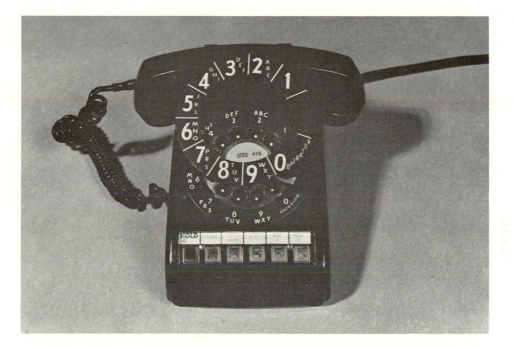

Fig. XV-2.   Miles Kimball large number telephone dial. The enlarged numbers on the dial shown are 10.3M size. Black on white dials are available from other sources.

6. Where distance requirements are a consideration, such as notes to be used in a speech, large type can be very useful to a person who might otherwise read normal size type at a very close distance.

7. Elderly people who reject the decreased working distance required by a low vision aid, or the use of a telescopic spectacle may be willing to accept large print books and should be advised of their availability. It is advisable to have one of these books in the office to test and demonstrate their ability to read them.

B. Telephone dials

1. Large number telephone dials are available and can be pasted over the normal numerals and letters of the regular dial (see Figure XV-2).

2. Since it is often inconvenient to use relative distance magnification with a telephone dial, this type of magnification is very convenient.

C. Playing cards

1. Jumbo and large pip playing cards permit the cards to be seen on the table under circumstances where reducing the working distance would be very impractical (see Figure XV-3).

2. Sometimes contrast and illumination play a large role. A combination of a dull green table cover and a strong lamp along with the jumbo or large pip playing cards may solve the problem.

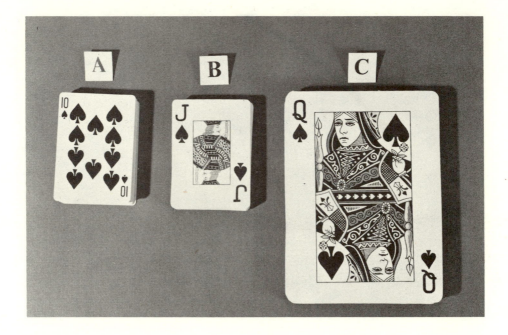

Fig. XV-3.   Playing cards.
  A.   Standard, 6.3M size digits and letters.
  B.   Large pip, 10M size digits and letters. Note that the central area is minified compared to the standard.
  C.   Jumbo, 12M size digits and letters. Note that the central area is also enlarged compared to the standard.

Stands

A. General

Relative distance magnification may require placing books or other material at an unusually close working distance which may be tiring to the arms. Furthermore minute variations in this close distance may produce significant blurring and therefore holding the material at a constant distance becomes very important. The majority of low vision patients are elderly and may have other handicaps resulting in hand tremors and the inability to sustain the weight of a large print book for any length of time. Stands are very useful for solving these problems and may be essential for utilization of a magnifying aid.

B. Reading stands

Ordinary reading stands (see Figure XV-4) may be sufficient in some cases. They hold the material steady and upright so that the reader is not forced to bend over a table.

C. Table easels

In many instances it is necessary to hold the material upright and above the table so that the book is directly in front of the patient's eyes. For this purpose and for writing, a table easel with an adjustable shelf is quite useful (see Figure XV-5).

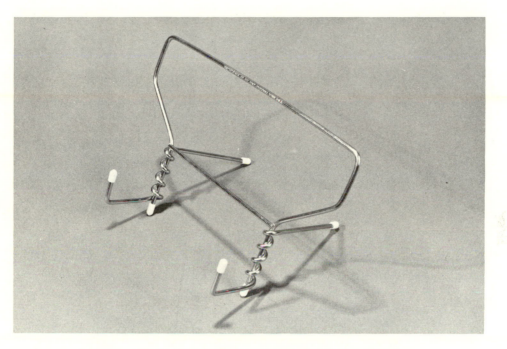

Fig. XV-4.   Folding wire book stand.

D. Piano music stands

Special stands for piano music are available from the American Printing House for the Blind. These permit a shortened working distance.

   1. A simple stand is made for upright pianos (see Figure XV-6).

   2. The Gore Reading Stand may be adapted for grand or spinet type pianos (see Figure XV-7).

E. Music stands

Regular music stands or adaptations of them can be used to hold material for typing, reading, lecturing, etc.

F. Other stands

Many stands, tables, etc., have been adapted for low vision patients. Among these are bed stands, hospital bed tables, drafting tables, etc.

Writing Aids

A. General

Numerous writing aids are available to provide magnification, contrast enhancement and tactual clues.

B. Typewriters

These are available with large type and/or large lettered keys. Keys can also be "Braille" coded. New black or special carbon ribbons should be used to produce maximum contrast. Frequent ribbon changes, type character cleanings and general servicing are necessary to maintain optimal legibility.

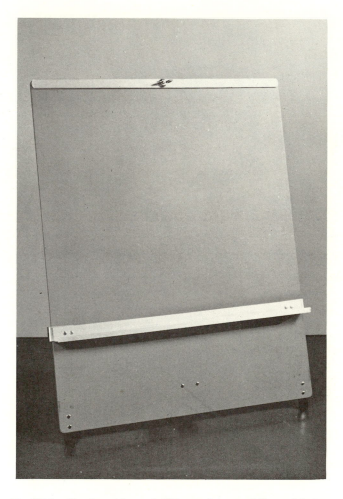

Fig. XV-5.   Testrite table easel. This stand is especially useful since the shelf can be placed at any position from the top to the bottom of the back and the stand angle can be varied 90 degrees.

C. Implements

    1. Because of the obvious disadvantages of writing in a severely reduced working space, implements that provide magnification and enhanced contrast are often preferred. Black felt and nylon tip pens afford heavy strokes and good contrast. Where pencil is needed, a soft lead (#4 or higher) can be used. Art supply stores are good sources for a variety of these special pens and pencils.

    2. Where reduced working space is unavoidable, stubby pens and short pencils can be used.

D. Paper

    1. Dull paper is preferable to glossy.

    2. Ruled paper with wide spaces and heavy lines is available from the American Printing House

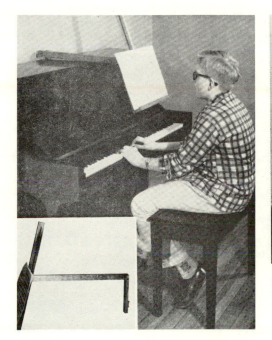

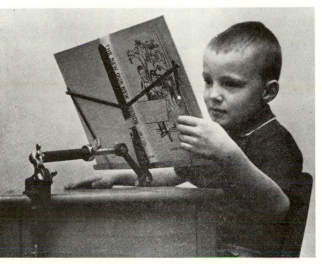

Fig. XV-7. Gore Reading Stand. Photo courtesy of The American Printing House for the Blind.

Fig. XV-6. Music stand for an upright piano. Photo courtesy of The American Printing House for the Blind.

for the Blind (see Figure XV-8). For those requiring tactual clues for writing straight, raised line paper is available from the same source.

E. Stencils

Stencils (line guides) are available or can be custom made in many forms (see Figure XV-9). They are particularly useful for bank checks or as signature guides.

Blind Aids

A. General

Most partially-sighted patients are unaware of the many aids available for use *without* vision, since these are distributed primarily by organizations for the blind. Such devices may have a great utility for people having some reduction of visual ability. Anyone working in this field should thoroughly familiarize himself with the aids and appliances catalogue of the American Foundation for the Blind. Often useful devices can be found in local stores.

B. Sewing aids

Some of the more useful devices are:

    1. Self-threading needles (see Figure XV-10)

    2. Needle threaders (see Figure XV-11).

        a. Hand needles

        b. Sewing machine

    3. Colored and large head pins

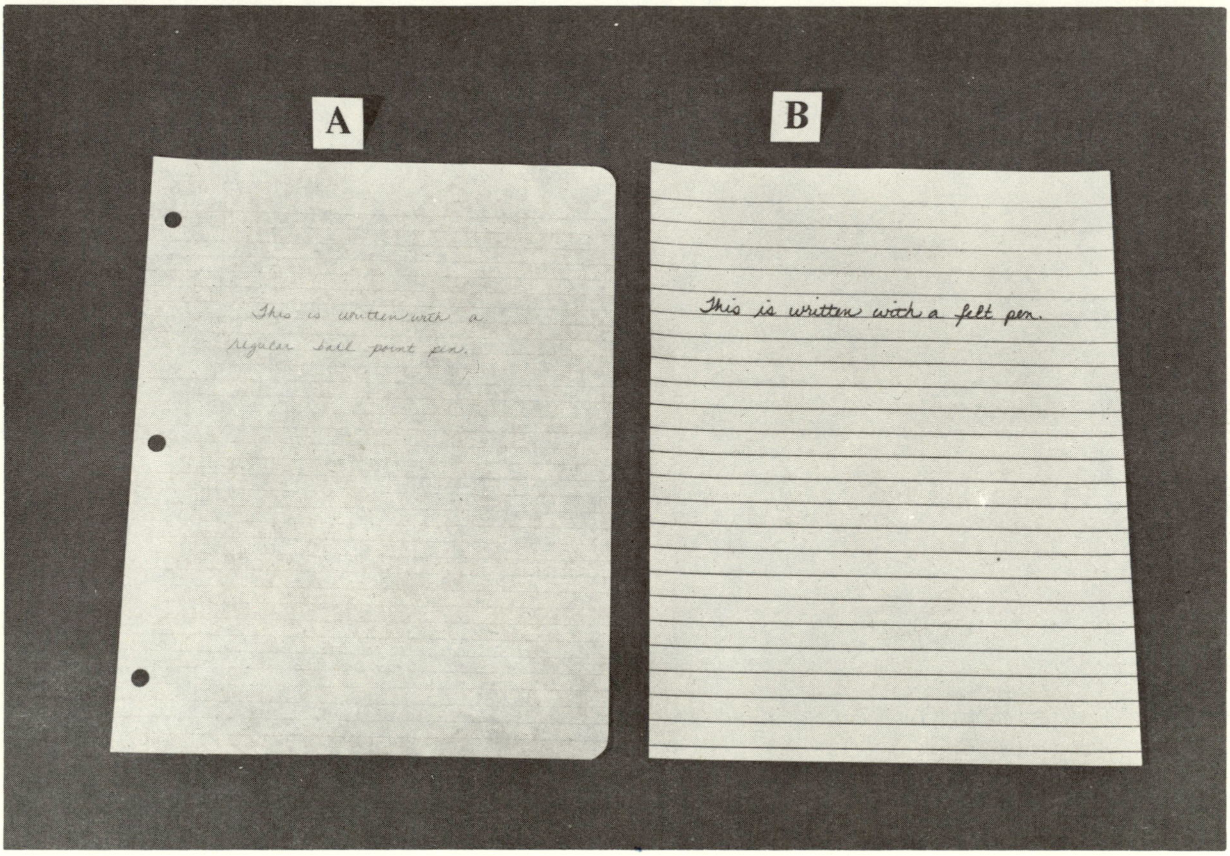

Fig. XV-8.   *Heavy lined paper.*
  A.   Ordinary lined paper with writing produced with a regular blue ball point pen.
  B.   Heavy lined, wide space paper with writing produced with a black, thin felt, pen. The improvement in contrast is striking.

    4. Tape measures
       a. Braille
       b. Staple coded (see Figure XV-12)
  C. Kitchen utensils
     1. Raised marked measuring utensils
     2. Shredders incorporating a catch bowl (see Figure XV-13)
     3. Food cutting guides (see Figure XV-14)
     4. Raised stove markings
     5. Dark water glasses
     6. Etc.
  D. Braille watches and timers

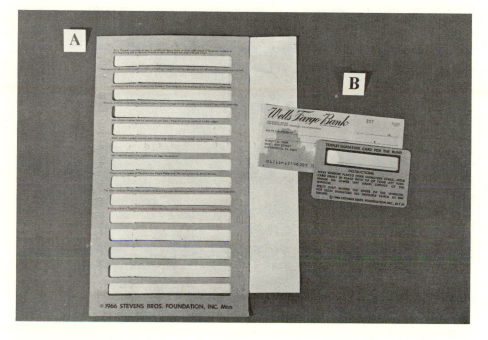

Fig. XV-9.   Stencil line guides.
   A.   Writing guide.
   B.   Signature guide. Check guides can be made to match a specific check size and provide correct slots for all writing required.

E. Talking Books
   1. Books are available on recordings and tapes through the Library of Congress without charge to the visually handicapped. Machines to play them are also available without charge. The American Foundation for the Blind Directory lists the source of these books in each state.

   2. Recordings for the Blind will make tapes, on request, of textbooks for college students who require these aids.

   3. It is not unusual for a person to use an optical aid for their correspondence or the daily newspaper, but to rely on Talking Books for pleasure reading or prolonged periods of study.

Mobility Aids
A. General
In recent years special curricula have been offered at various colleges to provide mobility instructors (peripatologists). They have been especially trained to teach the visually handicapped the use of special techniques and aids to promote mobility and independence.
The techniques usually involve the use of the other senses, memory, and reasoning. The principal aid in use at this time is the long cane.

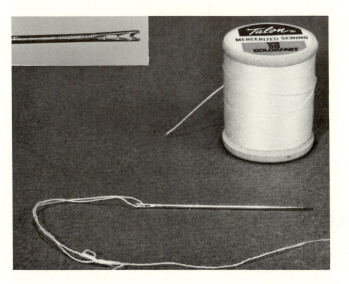

Fig. XV-10.   "Self-threading" needles. The thread is pushed through the knotch at the top rather than being inserted through the eye.

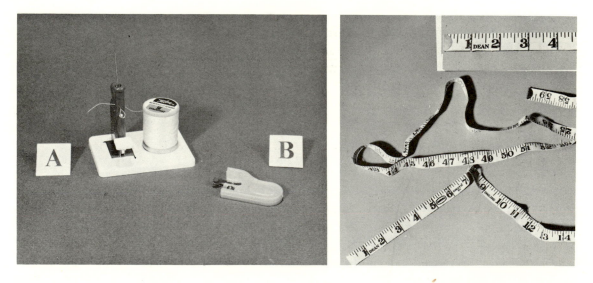

Fig. XV-11.   Automatic needle threaders.
A.   For manual needles.
B.   For sewing machine needles.

Fig. XV-12.   Staple coded tape measure. A single staple is oriented vertically at each inch mark. A horizontal staple is added, at the top, every six inches. A third staple is added at each foot mark.

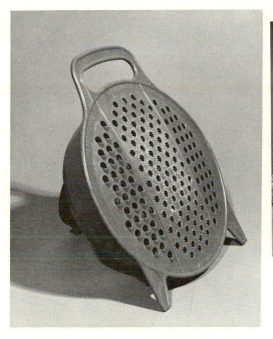

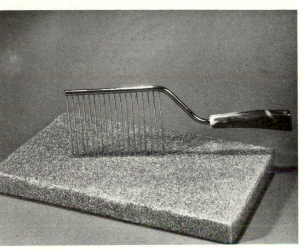

Fig. XV-14.   *Food cutting guide.*

Fig. XV-13.   *Shredder with attached catch bowl.*

B. Long canes

The long cane (see Figure XV-15) developed by Richard Hoover in the 1940's, is radically different from the orthopedic cane previously used. This cane has no support function but rather has been designed to efficiently sense the environment.

Long canes are available in varying lengths and materials as well as collapsible and non-collapsible designs. With proper training this cane allows the user to walk erect at a normal pace in strange environments without the use of vision.

Some low vision patients find canes helpful in certain circumstances where their vision is inadequate such as unfavorable illumination. Others use white canes (often orthopedic style) as identification and warning to sighted travelers. Since the cane is used intermittently, partially-sighted users prefer the collapsible models.

C. Newer developments

1. Various remote sensors have been designed or proposed and are being investigated, which allow the user to assess the environment beyond the reach of a cane. The devices also allow assessment of areas of the environment not normally surveyed with a cane (e.g. areas above waist level).

Among these devices are radar-like systems using laser or ultrasonic beams with the return information converted to tactual or auditory signals. Thus far, these have been made in the forms of canes, eyeglasses, and hand held probes.

2. In recent years research and development programs have been directed toward vision substitute systems. These systems receive visual information which is converted electronically to

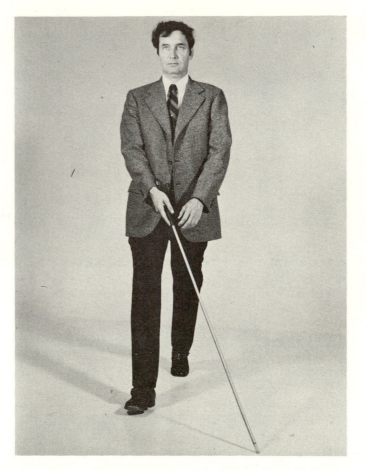

Fig. XV-15.   Walking with a long cane. The cane is rhythmically swung from side to side along the path. In the photo, the cane is "clearing" the area prior to the left foot entering it. As the left foot advances, the cane is swung to the right to "clear" that area prior to the next advance of the right foot.

another sensory modality which in turn transmits this information to the brain. The brain then interprets this as visual information.

   a. Bach-Y-Rita et al. (1969) have developed and tested a system that utilizes a television camera and tactile stimulation of the skin of the torso to produce "visual" perception in totally blind individuals.

   b. Bliss and Crane (1969) have designed the Optacon, a miniature camera-probe which reads letters and numbers and converts them to vibrations on the finger which also results in "visual" perceptions.

3. Brindley and Lewin (1968), as well as other groups, have been researching the feasibility of by-passing the body's sensory modalities and feeding electronic impulses directly into the visual cortex to produce patterns of phosphenes.

Chapter 16

Sources of Low Vision Aids

General

The more successful practitioners in the low vision field seem to maintain the approach of prescribing those devices which solve the patient's problems regardless of the disadvantages inherent in the aids. There is no single aid or type of aid which is a panacea. While it is possible to assemble a small number of aids which will be useful to a majority of low vision patients, it is also true that many patients' needs will not be fully met with this limited approach.

If the eclectic and pragmatic approach is to be followed, success will be somewhat dependent upon the prescriber's knowledge of the various aids and their availability. Many low vision aids are not primarily designed or manufactured for the low vision patient and thus are not necessarily available through the normal ophthalmic supply channels. Hence, it is imperative that each low vision practitioner develop and maintain his own catalogues of low vision aids and their sources. Since aids and sources are continually changing, these catalogues must be revised frequently.

This chapter is an attempt to formulate a list of low vision aids and sources familiar to the authors. It must be realized that any such list will not include all aids available nor will it be completely accurate relative to those that are included, if for no other reason than the lag between writing and publication.

Social Agencies

The low vision practitioner should be aware of the services and benefits offered by federal agencies such as the Veterans Administration, the Social Security Administration, and the Internal Revenue Service. Most state social service and education departments and their local counterparts maintain services for the visually handicapped. There are also frequently private local agencies offering services.

Among the various services offered by both public and private agencies are: financial assistance, vocational training and counselling, psychological counselling, educational assistance, medical and optometric care, blind rehabilitation, etc.

The American Foundation for the Blind publishes a directory listing both public and private agencies in each state.

LOW VISION AIDS, OPTICAL

	Illumination Controls	Loupes and Lenses, Clip-On	Loupes, Headborne	Magnifiers, Hand	Magnifiers, Stand (focusable)	Magnifiers, Stand (non-focusable)	Microscopic and Rx Lenses	Projection Magnifiers	Special Frames	Telescopes, Clip-On	Telescopes, Hand-held	Telescopes, Headborne	Telescopes, Prescription	Testing Equipment	COMMENTS
The Albert Aloe Co. 805 Locust Street St. Louis, Mo.										•					
American Bifocal Co., Inc. 1440 St. Clair Avenue Cleveland, Ohio							•								Volk-Conoid Lenses
American Optical Co., Inc. 14 Mechanic Street Southbridge, Mass. 01550		•					•							•	Request information from: Lens Products Dept. 4617
Amoriex-Ward Instrument Corp. 322 Belleville Pike North Arlington, New Jersey 07032		•	•												
Apex Specialties Co. 1115 Douglas Avenue Providence, R. I. 02904	•	•	•	•	•	•	•								
Apollo Lasers, Inc. 6365 Arizona Circle Los Angeles, Calif. 90045								•							Closed-circuit television
Armorlite, Inc. 727 S. Main Street Burbank, Calif. 91506							•								
Bausch & Lomb, Inc. 635 St. Paul Street Rochester, New York 14602	•	•	•	•	•	•	•					•		•	

LOW VISION AIDS, OPTICAL

	Illumination Controls	Loupes and Lenses, Clip-On	Loupes, Headborne	Magnifiers, Hand	Magnifiers, Stand (focusable)	Magnifiers, Stand (non-focusable)	Microscopic and Rx Lenses	Projection Magnifiers	Special Frames	Telescopes, Clip-On	Telescopes, Hand-held	Telescopes, Headborne	Telescopes, Prescription	Testing Equipment	COMMENTS
Behr Manufacturing Co. 744 E. Wisconsin Avenue Oconomowoc, Wisconsin		●													
Berg Industries Steady-Vue Division 3376 West First Street Los Angeles, Calif. 90004									●						Binocular attachment
Bernell Corporation 316 South Eddy Street South Bend, Indiana 46617	●	●	●	●	●	●	●			●	●			●	
Bolsey Research & Development Windsor Park P. O. Box 248 Hartsdale, New York 10530							●								Fresnel Lenses
Brower, Archibald D. Co. 3101 Pierce Street San Francisco, Calif. 94123			●						●			●			
B. S. A. Industries 2697 Cleveland Ave. Columbus, Ohio 43211							●							●	High add plastic bifocals
Burton Manufacturing Co. 7922 Haskell Avenue Van Nuys, Calif. 91406	●		●	●											

LOW VISION AIDS, OPTICAL

	Illumination Controls	Loupes and Lenses, Clip-On	Loupes, Headborne	Magnifiers, Hand	Magnifiers, Stand (focusable)	Magnifiers, Stand (non-focusable)	Microscopic and Rx Lenses	Projection Magnifiers	Special Frames	Telescopes, Clip-On	Telescopes, Hand-held	Telescopes, Headborne	Telescopes, Prescription	Testing Equipment	COMMENTS
Bushnell 2828 E. Foothill Blvd. Pasadena, Calif.											●				
Colonial Optical Co., Inc. 1954 S. La Cienega Blvd. Los Angeles, Calif.	●		●	●	●						●	●			
Covington Plating Works, Inc. 331 Pike Street Covingtom, Ky. 41011	●				●										Adisco illuminated magnifier
Designs for Vision, Inc. 40 East 21st Street New York, N. Y. 10010	●					●	●	●	●		●		●	●	Feinbloom lenses and charts
Donegan Optical Co., Inc. 1405 Kansas Kansas City, Mo. 64127		●	●	●		●									
Eberson Enterprises P. O. Box 5516 Pasadena, Calif.	●														Visor
Edmund Scientific Co. 602 Edscorp Bldg. Barrington, N. J. 08007	●	●	●	●	●	●	●			●	●	●			
The Ednalite Corporation 210 North Water Street Peekskill, N. Y. 10566	●				●										Illuminated Stand Magnifier

LOW VISION AIDS, OPTICAL

	Illumination Controls	Loupes and Lenses, Clip-On	Loupes, Headborne	Magnifiers, Hand	Magnifiers, Stand (focusable)	Magnifiers, Stand (non-focusable)	Microscopic and Rx Lenses	Projection Magnifiers	Special Frames	Telescopes, Clip-On	Telescopes, Hand-held	Telescopes, Headborne	Telescopes, Prescription	Testing Equipment	COMMENTS
Edroy Products Co., Inc. 130 West 29th Street New York, N. Y. 10001	•	•	•	•	•	•									
Efron, Marvin O. D. 1205 D. Avenue West Columbia, S. C. 29169						•									Visolette Dome Magnifier
Electro-Optix, Inc. 35-12 Crescent Street Long Island City, N. Y. 11106	•			•											Pocket Illuminated Magnifier
Fostoria-Fannon, Inc. 1200 North Main Street Fostoria, Ohio 44830	•					•									Illuminated Stand Magnifier, Various lamps
The Good-Lite Company 7426 W. Madison Street Forest Park, Ill. 60130														•	Acuity charts
Hamblin, Theodore, Limited 15 Wigmore Street London W1, England							•		•				•	•	Bier lenses
House of Vision 135-37 N. Wabash Avenue Chicago, Ill. 60602	•	•	•	•	•	•	•			•	•		•	•	

LOW VISION AIDS, OPTICAL

	Illumination Controls	Loupes and Lenses, Clip-On	Loupes, Headborne	Magnifiers, Hand	Magnifiers, Stand (focusable)	Magnifiers, Stand (non-focusable)	Microscopic and Rx Lenses	Projection Magnifiers	Special Frames	Telescopes, Clip-On	Telescopes, Hand-held	Telescopes, Headborne	Telescopes, Prescription	Testing Equipment	COMMENTS
Jadow, B. & Sons 53 West 23rd Street New York, N. Y. 10010		●													Ary Loupes
Keeler Optical Prod. Inc. 456 Parkway Lawrence Park Industrial Dist. Broomall, Pa. 19008	●	●		●	●	●	●		●		●	●	●		
Kono Manufacturing Co., Inc. 69-24 49th Avenue Woodside, New York 11377	●	●							●			●			Ptosis crutch Moveable shields, Hemianopsia mirrors, etc.
The Lighthouse The N. Y. Assn. for the Blind Low Vision Services 111 East 59th Street New York, N. Y. 10022	●	●		●	●	●	●			●	●	●		●	Sloan Magnifier; I-Gard and COIL magnifiers
Magna-Add, Incorporated 150 East Broad St., Suite 706 Columbus, Ohio 43215		●													Clip-on Bifocal
McLeod Optical Co., Inc. 357 Westminster Street Providence, Rhode Island				●		●	●							●	I-Gard and COIL magnifiers
May Manufacturing Corp. P.O. Box 437 7 Barnabas Road Marion, Mass. 02738	●	●	●						●						Stenopaic Spectacles

LOW VISION AIDS, OPTICAL

	Illumination Controls	Loupes and Lenses, Clip-On	Loupes, Headborne	Magnifiers, Hand	Magnifiers, Stand (focusable)	Magnifiers, Stand (non-focusable)	Microscopic and Rx Lenses	Projection Magnifiers	Special Frames	Telescopes, Clip-On	Telescopes, Hand-held	Telescopes, Headborne	Telescopes, Prescription	Testing Equipment	COMMENTS
New Era Optical Co. 17 N. Wabash Avenue Chicago, Illinois 6069	•	•	•	•	•	•	•			•	•	•		•	
Nusinov, Charles & Sons, Inc. 1404 E. Baltimore Street Baltimore, Md. 21231		•													Ary Loupes
Nu-Vue Visor Company P. O. Box 757 Fairhope, Alabama 36532	•														Visor
Ocular Instruments Co. P. O. Box 1787 Los Gatos, California 95030											•			•	Emoskop 3×
Opaque Systems Ltd. 100 Taft Avenue Hempstead, N. Y. 11550					•			•							Opaque Projector and Closed circuit television
Optical Sciences Group, Inc. 2201 Webster Street San Francisco, Cal. 94115				•				•							Fresnel lenses and prisms
Pelco Sales Inc. 351 E. Alondra Blvd. Gardena, CA. 90248								•							Closed circuit television
E. W. Pike & Co., Inc. 577 Pennsylvania Avenue Elizabeth, N. J. 07207	•						•								

LOW VISION AIDS, OPTICAL

	Illumination Controls	Loupes and Lenses, Clip-On	Loupes, Headborne	Magnifiers, Hand	Magnifiers, Stand (focusable)	Magnifiers, Stand (non-focusable)	Microscopic and Rx Lenses	Projection Magnifiers	Special Frames	Telescopes, Clip-On	Telescopes, Hand-held	Telescopes, Headborne	Telescopes, Prescription	Testing Equipment	COMMENTS
Policoff Laboratories 68 S. Franklin Street Wilkes-Barre, Pa.							●							●	
Prentiss Precision Div. of Transcontinental Sales Co. 1608 W. Pico Blvd. Los Angeles, CA. 90015	●	●	●	●	●	●					●	●			
Ravadge Instruments 731 Biddle Road Glen Burnie, Md. 21063	●			●											Sloan Illuminated Magnifiers
Selsi Company, Inc. 40 Veterans Blvd. Carlstadt, N. J. 07072	●	●	●	●	●	●				●	●	●			
Shuron-Continental 40 Humbolt Street Rochester, N. Y. 14609							●								High add Ultex Bifocal
Superior Optical Company 1500 S. Hope Street Los Angeles, CA. 90015	●														Typoscope
Swift Instruments, Inc. 952 Dorchester Avenue Boston, Mass. 02125 or 1190 North 4th San Jose, CA. 95106			●	●	●						●				

LOW VISION AIDS, OPTICAL

	Illumination Controls	Loupes and Lenses, Clip-On	Loupes, Headborne	Magnifiers, Hand	Magnifiers, Stand (focusable)	Magnifiers, Stand (non-focusable)	Microscopic and Rx Lenses	Projection Magnifiers	Special Frames	Telescopes, Clip-On	Telescopes, Hand-held	Telescopes, Headborne	Telescopes, Prescription	Testing Equipment	COMMENTS
Telesight, Inc. 1418 East 88th Street Brooklyn, N. Y. 11236	●	●	●	●	●	●			●	●		●			
Universal Ophthalmic Prods. P. O. Box 3144 Houston, Texas 77001							●								Temporary Cataract Lenses
Visorette 3141 E. California Blvd. Pasadena, California (P. O. Box 5185)	●														Visor
Visualtek 1840 Lincoln Blvd. Santa Monica, CA. 90404								●							Closed circuit television
Watchemoket Optical Co., Inc. 232 West Exchange St. Providence, R. I. 02903	●								●						
Western Optical 1200 Mercer Street Seattle, Washington 98109	●	●	●	●	●	●				●		●		●	
X-Pert 6563 Mammoth Ave. Van Nuys, CA. 91401								●							Closed curcuit television
Yorktowne Optical Co. 469 W. Market Street York, Pa. 17404	●														Slip-in Wrap-around Sunshade

LOW VISION AIDS, OPTICAL

	Illumination Controls	Loupes and Lenses, Clip-On	Loupes, Headborne	Magnifiers, Hand	Magnifiers, Stand (focusable)	Magnifiers, Stand (non-focusable)	Microscopic and Rx Lenses	Projection Magnifiers	Special Frames	Telescopes, Clip-On	Telescopes, Hand-held	Telescopes, Headborne	Telescopes, Prescription	Testing Equipment	COMMENTS
Younger Manufacturing Co. 3788 S. Broadway Place Los Angeles, CA. 90007	●				●										
Zeiss, Carl 444 Fifth Avenue New York, N. Y. 10018	●	●	●			●	●				●		●	●	

LOW VISION AIDS, NON-OPTICAL

	Braille	Large Type	Recordings	Information	Avocational Aids	Kitchen Aids	Mobility Aids	Music Aids	Reading Aids	School Aids	Sewing Aids	Vocational Aids	Writing Aids	COMMENTS
American Foundation for the Blind, Inc. 15 West 16th Street New York, N. Y. 10011	•	•		•	•	•	•	•		•	•	•	•	
American Library Assoc. 50 East Huron Street Chicago, Illinois 60611	•	•	•	•					•	•				Catalogue of sources only
American Printing House for the Blind 1839 Frankfort Avenue Louisville, Kentucky	•		•	•	•			•	•	•			•	
Better Vision Institute, Inc. 230 Park Avenue New York, N. Y. 10017		•												List of large type producers
Betty Crocker General Mills, Inc. Minneapolis, Minnesota			•											Recorded recipes
Braille Institute of America 741 North Vermont Ave. Los Angeles, California	•		•	•	•	•	•	•	•	•	•	•	•	
G. K. Hall & Co. 70 Lincoln Street Boston, Mass. 02111		•												
Industrial Home for the Blind 20 Park Avenue Brooklyn, New York				•										

LOW VISION AIDS, NON-OPTICAL

	Braille	Large Type	Recordings	Information	Avocational Aids	Kitchen Aids	Mobility Aids	Music Aids	Reading Aids	School Aids	Sewing Aids	Vocational Aids	Writing Aids	COMMENTS
Keith Jennison Books Franklin Watts, Inc. 575 Lexington Avenue New York, N. Y. 10022		●												
Large Print, Ltd. 505 Pearl Street Buffalo, New York 14202		●												Large print booklist
Library of Congress Division for the Blind & Physically Handicapped Washington, D. C.	●	●	●	●										
The Lighthouse The N. Y. Assoc. for the Blind Low Vision Services 111 East 59th Street New York, N. Y. 10022		●		●					●				●	
The Microfilm Co. of Calif. 1977 S. Los Angeles Street Los Angeles, CA. 90011		●												
Miles Kimball 41 West Eighth Avenue Oshkosh, Wisconsin 54901		●			●									Phone dials and playing cards
National Aid to the Visually Handicapped 3201 Balboa Street San Francisco, California		●							●					Large print books and book stand

LOW VISION AIDS, NON-OPTICAL

	Braille	Large Type	Recordings	Information	Avocational Aids	Kitchen Aids	Mobility Aids	Music Aids	Reading Aids	School Aids	Sewing Aids	Vocational Aids	Writing Aids	COMMENTS
National Society for the Prevention of Blindness 16 East 40th Street New York, N. Y. 10016				●										
New York Times Large Type Weekly 229 West 43rd Street New York, N. Y. 10036		●												
Pacific Gas & Electric Co. 245 Market Street San Francisco, California						●								Special aids for kitchen ranges
Contact local Utility Co. outside of P.G.&E. area														
Readers Digest Pleasantville, N. Y. 10570		●												Large type edition
Recording for the Blind 215 East 58th Street New York, N. Y. 10022			●											
Stanwix House Publishers 1306 Highland Building Pittsburg, Pennsylvania		●												
Testrite Instrument Co., Inc. 135 Monroe Street Newark, New Jersey 07105									●					Table easel

LOW-VISION AIDS, NON-OPTICAL

	Braille	Large Type	Recordings	Information	Avocational Aids	Kitchen Aids	Mobility Aids	Music Aids	Reading Aids	School Aids	Sewing Aids	Vocational Aids	Writing Aids	COMMENTS
Xerox Corporation Box 330 Department XB Grand Central Station New York, N. Y. 10017		●												

References

Abrams, Bernard (1955), Correcting nystagmus with corneal lenses, Optom. Weekly, 46 (20): 809-812.

Adams, Anthony, Allan N. Freid and Edwin B. Mehr (1974), to be published.

Asher, H. (1970), Effect on vergence of a forward movement of a spectacle lens—a classical fallacy, Optom. Weekly, 61 (33): 719-721.

Bach-y-Rita, Paul, Carter C. Collins, Benjamin White, Frank A. Saunders, Lawrence Scadden, and Robert Blomberg (1969), A tactile vision substitution system, Am. J. of Optom. and Arch. Am. Acad. of Optom., 46 (2): 109-111.

Bechtold, Edwin W. (1953), An improved system of wide angle magnifying spectacles, Opt. J. and Rev. of Optom., 90 (22): 35.

Benjamin, J. Malvern Jr. (1968), A review of the Veterans Administration blind guidance project, Bull. of Prosthetics Research, Wash., D. C., Veterans Administration, Spring.

Berne, Eric (1964), Games People Play, Grove Press.

Bettman, J. W., and G. S. McNair (1939), A contact-lens-telescopic system, Amer. J. Ophthal., 22 (1): 27-32.

Bier, Norman (1970), Correction of Subnormal Vision, 2nd ed. New York, Appleton-Century Crofts.

Blasch, Donald and Loyal E. Apple (1966), Severe visual impairments, Long Cane News Letter, 2 (1): 1-4 (Published by Peripatology Program, Boston College).

Bliss, F. C. and H. D. Crane (1969), Touch as a means of communication, J. of the Stanford Research Institute, Feature Issue, 5: 2-15.

Borish, Irvin M. (1970), Clinical Refraction, 3rd ed. Chicago, Professional Press.

Brazelton, Frank A. (1964), Aid for the partially-sighted—the dimensions of the problem, J. of Calif. Optom. Assn., 32 (6): 22.

————(1969), Magnification in microscopic lenses, Am. J. Optom. and Arch. Am. Acad. Optom., 46 (4): 304-308.

Brindley, G. S. and W. S. Lewin (1968), Sensations produced by electrical stimulation of the visual cortex, J. of Physiol., 196: 479-493.

Cholden, Louis S. (1958), A Psychiatrist Works With Blindness. New York, American Foundation for the Blind.

Cowen, Emory L., Rita B. Underberg, Ronald T. Verrilla and Frank S. Benham (1961), Adjustment to Visual Disability in Adolescence, New York, American Foundation for the Blind.

Davis, John (1969), Some Simple Spectacle Aids for Low Vision—Structure and Performance, Paper presented at American Academy of Optometry Annual Meeting, Dec.

————(1970), Letter communication.

————(1971), Letter communication.

Ellerbrock, Vincent J. (1960), in Hirsch, Monroe J. and Ralph E. Wick, Vision of the Aging Patient. Chapt. 10, pp. 174-201, Phila., Chilton Co.

Englemann, Otto R. (1961), Subjective pupillary distance measurement, Optom. Weekly 52 (39).

Faye, Eleanor E. (1970), The Low Vision Patient, New York, Grune and Stratton.

Feinbloom, William (1960), Lecture: Subnormal Vision and Clinic, Post Graduate Course at Am. Acad. of Optom. Meeting, San Francisco, Dec.

Filderman, Irving P. (1959), The telecon lens for the partially-sighted, Am. J. Optom. and Arch. Am. Acad. of Optom., 36 (3): 135-136.

Flom, Merton C. (1966), New concepts on visual acuity, Optom. Weekly, 57 (28): 63-68.

————, Frank W. Weymouth, and Daniel Kahneman (1963), Visual resolution and contour interaction, J. of Opt. Soc. of Am., 53 (9): 1026-1032.

Fonda, Gerald (1965), Management of the Patient with Subnormal Vision. St. Louis, C. V. Mosby Co.

Freid, Allan N. (1973), Unpublished paper.

Genensky, Sam M., P. Baran, H. L. Moshin, and H. Steingold, (1968), A Closed Circuit TV System for the Visually Handicapped, Santa Monica, The Rand Corporation, RM-5672-RC, Aug.

Genensky, Sam M. (1973), Binoculars: A Long-Ignored Aid for the Partially Sighted, Santa Monica, The Rand Corporation, R-1402-HEW, Nov.

Glass, Edward J. (1970), The social psychological adjustment to low residual vision, Proceedings of the Low Vision Conference, San Francisco, U. S. Office of Education.

Goldish, Louis H. and Michael H. Marx (1973), The visually impaired as a market for sensory aids and services; part two—aids and services for partially sighted persons, New Outlook for the Blind, 67 (7): 289-296.

Goodlaw, Edward I. (1968), Homework for low vision patients, Am. J. Optom. and Arch. Am. Acad. Optom., 45 (8): 532-538.

Gregg, James R. and Gordon G. Heath (1964), The Eye and Sight. Boston, D. C. Heath and Co.

Grosvenor, Theodore P. (1963), Contact Lens Theory and Practice. Chicago, The Professional Press.

Guth, Sylvester K. (1957), Effect of age on visibility, Am. J. of Optom. and Arch. of Am. Acad. of Optom., 34 (9): 463-477.

Haley, Jay (1963), Strategies of Psychotherapy. New York, Grune and Stratton.

Hirsch, Monroe J. (1964), Introduction, J. of Calif. Optom. Assn., 32 (6): 5.

Howard, Norman H. (1959), The N. H. Howard Card., 338 Cajon St., Redlands, Calif.

Igersheimer, J. (1919), Graefe's Arch. of Ophth., 100: 357.

Industrial Home for the Blind (1957), Optical Aids Service—Survey on 500 Cases—March 1953 to December 1955. New York, Industrial Home for the Blind.

Jenkins, Francis A. and Harvey E. White (1957), Fundamentals of Optics, 3rd ed. New York, McGraw-Hill Book Co., p. 181.

Jessen, George N. (1969), High adds in new form, Am. J. of Optom. and Arch. Am. Acad. of Optom., 46 (8): 631-634.

Kahn, Harold A. and Helen B. Moorhead (1973), Statistics on Blindness in the Model Reporting Area 1969-1970. DHEW Publications No. (NIH) 73-427, U. S. Govt. Printing Office.

Kay, Leslie (1965), Ultrasonic mobility aids for the blind, Proceedings Rotterdam Mobility Research Conference, pp. 9-16.

Keller, Burton W. (1971), Light and the aging eyes, J. of Am. Optom. Assn., 42 (11): 1034-1037.

Koetting, Robert A. (1962), Unusual Management Considerations in Low Vision Practice, Paper delivered at National Optometric Conference Week, American Optometric Association, New Orleans, Louisiana.

Kollner, H. (1912), Die Storungen des Farbensinns. Berlin, S. Karger.

Korb, Donald (1972), Personal communication.

Kubler-Ross, Elizabeth (1969), On Death and Dying. New York, The MacMillan Company.

Lairy, Gabrielle-Catherine (1969), Problems in the adjustment of the visually impaired child, New Outlook for the Blind, 63 (2): 33-41.

Lavieri, M. and G. B. Wilson (1972), A portable closed circuit television aid for the partially-sighted, Am. J. of Optom. and Arch. Am. Acad. of Optom., 49 (2): 178-179.

Lebensohn, J. E. (1936), Scientific and practical considerations involved in the near-vision test with presentation of a practical and information near vision chart, Am. J. of Ophth., 19: 110.

Ludlam, W. M. (1960), Clinical experience with the contact lens telescope, Am. J. Optom. and Arch. Am. Acad. of Optom., 37 (7): 363-372.

Maltz, Maxwell (1960), Psycho-Cybernetics. Prentice Hall.

Mandell, Robert B. (1965), Contact Lens Practice, Basic and Advanced. Illinois, Chas. C. Thomas.

Mazow, B. (1958), The pupilens—a preliminary report, Contacto, Vol. 2, Sept: 128-131.

Mehr, Edwin B., Allan B. Frost, and Loyal E. Apple (1973), Experience with closed circuit television in the blind rehabilitation program of the Veterans Administration, Am. J. of Optom. and Arch. of Am. Acad. of Optom., 59 (6): 458-469.

Mehr, Edwin B., and Helen M. Mehr (1969), Psychological factors in working with partially sighted persons, J. Am. Optom. Assn. 40 (8): 842-846.

Mehr, Helen M., Edwin B. Mehr, and Carroll Ault (1970), Psychological aspects of low vision rehabilitation, Am. J. of Optom. and Arch. Am. Acad. of Optom., 47 (8): 605-612.

Morgan, Meredith W., Jr. (1962), Personal communication.

————(1972), Personal communication.

Neill, John C. (1953), The new clear image lens, Alumni Bulletin, P. S. C. O., 6 (6): 29-37.

Nooney, Thomas W. (1972), An optical approach to aid cerebral hemiplegics, Medical College of Virginia Quarterly, 8 (4): 274-277.

Policoff, William (1968), Personal communication.

Potts, A. M., D. Volk and S. W. West (1959), A television reader, Am. J. of Ophth., 47 (4).

Prentice, Charles F. (1897), The typoscope. The Keystone, Republished in Ophthalmic Lenses, Dioptric Formulae for Combined Cylindrical Lenses, The Prism-Dioptry and Other Papers by Charles F. Prentice. Philadelphia, The Keystone Publishing Company, 1907 (2d ed.).

———— and Edwin B. Mehr (1969), The typoscope, Am. J. of Optom. and Arch. Am. Acad. of Optom., 46 (11): 885-887.

Prince, Jack (1965), Typography for the low vision reader, Book Production Industry, Dec., Cleveland, Ohio, Penton Publishing Co.

Riley, Leo H. (1969), Low vision statistics, J. of Am. Optom. Assn., 40 (8): 820-827.

Rosenberg, Robert and D. Leonard Werner (1969), Nystagmus and low vision, J. of Am. Optom. Assn., 40 (8): 833-835.

Rosenbloom, Alfred A. (1966), Subnormal vision care: an analysis of clinic patients, Proceedings of the Conference on Aid to the Visually Limited, Washington, D. C., American Optometric Association, St. Louis.

———— (1969), The controlled-pupil contact lens in low vision problems, J. of Am. Optom. Assn., 40 (8): 836-840.

————(1970), Low Vision Aids in Borish, Irvin M., Clinical Refraction 3d ed. Chicago, Professional Press.

Schapero, Max, David Cline, and Henry William Hofstetter (1968), Dictionary of Visual Science, 2d ed., Phila., Chilton Book Co.

Schwartz, Robert E. (1960), Special report: Low Vision Center, Maryland Workshop for the Blind, Optom. Weekly, 51 (52): 2685-2687.

Sears, Francis W. (1948), Principles of Physics III, Optics, 3rd ed., Cambridge, Mass., Addison-Wesley Press, Inc., p. 131.

Sheard, Charles A. (1950), Ophthalmic Optics with Applications to Physiological Optics. The Year Book Publishers.

Simmons, R. E. (1966), Current ophthalmological attitudes toward rehabilitation of patients with loss of vision, New Outlook for the Blind, 60 (10): 299-301.

Sloan, Louise L. and Adelaide Habel (1957), New methods of rating and prescribing magnifiers for the partially blind, J. of Opt. Soc. of Am., 47 (8): 719-726.

Sloan, Louise L.and J. D. Brown (1963), Reading cards for selection of optical aids for the partially-sighted, Am. J. Ophth., 55 (6): 1187-1199.

Sloan, Louise L. (1971), Recommended Aids for the Partially Sighted, 2d ed., New York, National Society for the Prevention of Blindness.

Southall, James P. C. (1933a), Mirrors, Prisms, and Lenses, 3d ed. New York, The MacMillan Co., p. 452.

——— (1933b), Op. Cit., p. 459.

Stimson, R. L. (1957), Optical Aids for Low Acuity. Los Angeles, Braille Institute of America.

Sullivan, Henry Stack (1953), The Interpersonal Theory of Psychiatry. New York, W. W. Norton & Co.

Weed, C. A. (1968), Electronic image enlargement for the partially-sighted (a description of apparatus and preliminary results), Hartford Hospital Bull. 23 (1).

Weinstein, Edwin A. and Robert L. Kahn (1955), Denial of Illness. Springfield, Ill., Charles C. Thomas.

Weiss, Norman (1969), Management of the low vision patient with peripheral field loss, J. of Am. Optom. Assn., 40 (8): 830-832.

———(1972), An application of cemented prism with severe field loss, Am. J. of Optom. and Arch. Am. Acad. of Optom., 49 (3): 261-264.

Westheimer, Gerald (1957), The field of view of visual aids, Am. J. of Optom. and Arch. Am. Acad. of Optom., 34 (8): 430-438.

——— (1962), The visual world of the new contact lens wearer, J. of Am. Optom. Assn., 34 (2): 135-138.

Wild, Bradford W. (1968), A low vision lens design for reading, Optom. Weekly, 59 (15): 36-37.

INDEX

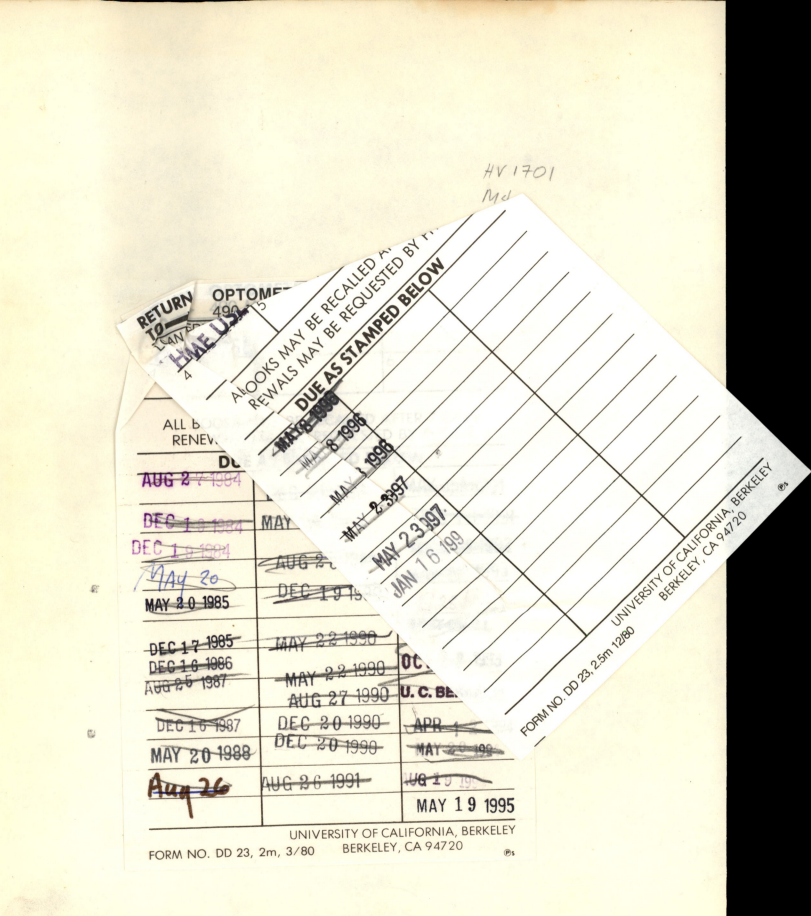

HV 1701
Md